He shall run and not
be weary and shall
walk and not faint

He shall run and not be weary and shall walk and not faint

Asdrúbal García

Library of Congress Control Number: 2016900653
ISBN: Hardcover   978-1-5065-1046-0
                   Softcover   978-1-5065-1045-3
                   eBook   978-1-5065-1044-6

The information, ideas, and suggestions in this book are not intended as a substitute for professional medical advice. Before following any suggestions contained in this book, you should consult your personal physician. Neither the author nor the publisher shall be liable or responsible for any loss or damage allegedly arising as a consequence of your use or application of any information or suggestions in this book.

The above biblical scriptures marked KJV are taken from The Holy Bible, King James version (version authorized). First published in 1611. Cited from the KJV Classic Reference Bible, Copyright © 1983 by Zondervan Coprporación.

Photo: Adilfa Ford from Don polo photography.

Print information available on the last page.

Rev. date: 14/01/2016

To order additional copies of this book, please contact:
Palibrio
1663 Liberty Drive,
Suite 200
Bloomington, IN 47403
Toll Free from the U.S.A 877.407.5847
Toll Free from Mexico 01.800.288.2243
Toll Free from Spain 900.866.949
From other International locations +1.812.671.9757
Fax: 01.812.355.1576
orders@palibrio.com
381399

PROLOGUE

Beginning to write a book is not easy. I've always desired to do it but I didn't know how? How to start? What topic? I just didn't know but I felt that I had to do it … until one day I had a spark inside me. Whipping up a smoothie of greens and other fruits and vegetables, a longtime friend of mine taught me some valuable insights of how important greens are in our lives … and this awakened an interest in me to eat healthier. It made me remember the time when I was a child and my mom taught me that with fruits and vegetables I could free myself from a bad stomach ache that I had suffered from for quite some time because of my poor eating habits.

So the name of the book came as part of my recent trip to Venezuela where I was trying to help my family eat healthier, show them I had lost weight in a healthy manner, and more importantly how I was able to free myself from so many sicknesses … every day as I made my green smoothies my family would say "you're turning me green with all your greens."

But by then end of my trip they started to feel better and healthier, and in only three weeks of sharing my smoothies with them, every morning they asked me for more greens. Later on Facebook, while chatting with them, they all started asking me for the recipe. Zulay Hurtado said that some family members didn't understand what it was all about, so I said better yet I'll write a book. I said it jokingly but then my cousin Adriana Torin had a dream that I had written this book and that same night I couldn't sleep thinking, what if I did it? What would I name it? Etc. Another friend of mine in Miami, Damaris Yajure (journalist) encouraged me saying she would help me write it and called me giving me ideas on how to start which was a big help. She said "your daughter already gave you the name, right!" Yanira said "Green, oh how I love you green" and ultimately my nephew Hector Enoc and said, "Uncle Asdrubal **'he shall run and not be weary and shall walk and not faint'** sounds better." I ended up keeping both names. I always wanted to make something more than just a recipe that would help purify and nourish our bodies both inside and out. I guarantee that what you're going to read from here on out will help you 100% in your health and overall success... as I write this book and share with you the secret of a healthier and more vitalizing life, I'm painting pictures, I sing, play the guitar, exercise, listen to music, chat with friends on Facebook...I'm very anxious but full of life and love, all of these things inspire me to do what I am doing.

I dedicate this book primarily to my mother who gave birth to me and taught me since I was a toddler to nourish my body especially with the famous 3in1(beets, carrot, and orange juice) and with a semi-vegetarian diet. I dedicate this book, also, to my family, my wife Gisela, children, grandchildren, including those who are more than just family, my best friends.

If it weren't for all of you and your inspiration I couldn't have accomplished this...

INTRODUCTION TO "GREEN, OH HOW I LOVE YOU GREEN"

As I said in the prologue this will be more than a recipe to lose weight healthily, the book includes various topics of motivation and an introduction to a healthy life like:

1- Attitude
2- Determination
3- Harmony in life
4- Health
5- Ingredients and properties of "Drubinlife"
6- "E-mail" for you to share
7- Presentation of Health
8- Symptoms that appear as we age and how to treat them

Attitude

Attitude is the key to success in life, 90% of all our success depends on our attitude, and the other 10% depends on the circumstances that surround you which you can't control. In our work there is much that is demanded of us and it depends on our attitude to accomplish it. For example, Peter has been working for a company for some time now so when he is asked to do something he just relies on his experience in the job and thinks that he doesn't need any explanations on how to do it, so he goes on as he always has. Later, Joe, who is new to the company and has a better attitude is asked to the same job and he does it in less time and better quality putting Peter's job at risk simply because of his attitude. Let's make it more understandable. To do things right, to be excited for yourself, even to start a new diet for yourself you need to have a good attitude or else you won't be motivated to continue with it. Do you remember the parable in the Bible of the good shepherd? (John 10:11-13) The salaried worker does his job out of obligation, the day the thieves come and rob the sheep he runs for his life. He doesn't defend them because they are not his. On the contrary, the real owner of the sheep defends them even to the point of laying down his own life. If you're not willing to defend your health with your own life and sacrifices, and you can't have a good attitude nothing will work until you change. If you're not willing to make the determination to look out for your own life nothing will work, including your relationship with your spouse, your diet, your projects, work, family, studies, etc. Of course 90% will depend on you, the other 10% we don't have any control over, but even so our attitude will be the vehicle that will take us to total triumph in all that we do.

All millionaires have achieved their success thanks to the good attitude and self-motivation they possess. Your life depends on you. Nobody will worry about you as much as you do! There is a biblical passage that says the second greatest commandment is to love your neighbor as yourself. No matter which religion you are, what we need to understand is that if we don't love ourselves enough to take care of this machine that takes us everywhere, which is our body, then who will?

We are willing to take care of our skin by bathing and using lotions and creams. We adorn ourselves with beautiful, nice, costly clothing. It's a lot like washing a car really good on the outside, making it shine with wax but never changing the oil, nor spark plugs, nor gas. One day it will break down and leave us stranded. Our vehicle was loaned to us to transport us everywhere, a perfect computer that connects and coordinates all of our feelings. Imagine letting in contaminating viruses to our computers or putting old dirty oil in your car's engine or putting soda in your gas tank instead of gasoline, or painting graffiti or breaking the windows out of your sacred temple which is your body... "What a disaster it would be, right"... well we have been doing exactly this, vandalizing our sacred bodies. We are the miracle of life but we have contaminated it with all the garbage that comes out in new television programs and advertisements. We know that anything in excess causes damage but we look for excuses as to why our bodies need them, like "our bodies need a certain amount of alcohol" so we store up enough for the whole year. We need some fat so we store up enough for 2 years and enough for 3 people, what are we doing? We prefer artificial soft drinks and diets without any vitamins, juices dirtied by carbonation contaminate our bodies and we say "well, we have to die of something." "That which doesn't kill makes one fat" and death by poor nutrition does not happen from one day to the next, it takes its time and kills slowly and the worst part of it is when you end up in the hospital without realizing why you are there. You don't remember that you yourself is the one to blame because of all the garbage that you put in your body. Why wait for a doctor to tell you that you have to stop eating this or that?

Some pay thousands of dollars and throw money away getting rid of fat with machinery that in one day they suck the fat from your body and sew you back up all new or you staple your stomach, lasers, and other procedures risking your life to only look better but continue eating the same stuff and following with the same traditions that you got in that position in the first place keeping the same attitude that with money everything is fixable...nooo!!! Our machine is dying off, the only vehicle that functioned perfectly in the beginning until we started to contaminate it.

We need to change our attitude and we will be able to enjoy better results and better health. But all of this will depend on your attitude. If these attitudes sound familiar to you, you need to make a change in your life. If you have tried everything and you feel like it's not worth trying anything else you need to change this belief and attitude to say; I want to try, I want to change, I want to get better, and that is how we evolve in our lives.

Determination

One must have courage to start any diet, undertake any undertaking, business or love relationship. I'm telling you that this will be more than a diet because you need to be good on all three of these points, if any of these three are lacking it can take you into depression and personal neglect.

We were and are created to resolve any situation that comes up in life. Depending on the determination we take, we will achieve change in our lives, destiny or future...courage is needed to make important decisions no matter if we win or lose. If we know that a certain path we take will yield us better results we need the courage to follow it. In the case of our health we know that putting more fruits and vegetables in our bodies that our organs will be better nourished.

Knowing that the results will be fabulous we can't hesitate or say tomorrow, next month, after Christmas, better yet when I'm making a little more money, or when I get a gym membership, or when my kids grow up, graduate or get married, or when I get a raise, or when I change jobs, when I move, when I have time, when summer starts, nooo!!! Enough with the excuses!!! The time is now!!! Enough will all the excuses and pretexts, today all the excuses died and now they don't exist in my vocabulary. Today I am determined to do it and nobody nor anything will stop me! Some dream of success others wake up and go looking for it. Either we do what will help our health or I stay in the same place making excuses. If this information is offensive to you and you are making excuses to not do this or read it judging what this book says, return the book or give it to someone who will utilize it...but if you decide to keep reading it until the end, the book and triumph is yours and that will make two of us winners.

Life is made up of "good decisions," "better decisions," and the appropriate or correct decision. "Which of the three do you think you are making?" Making the decision now to change your life for good? At least up until now I know that you have made a good decision to keep on reading the book, the better decision when you finish reading it and the most appropriate decision when you'll have decided to put into practice what we'll teach you here. Do you realize that? That's how you improve on making decisions in life. Even to get married and choose your future husband or wife, if you choose a good companion you will say "I made a good decision." You'll have children and live in harmony and mutual agreement (the better decision) ultimately they'll get married then come the grandchildren all happy then you'll say that was one of the best most appropriate correct decisions. When it comes to your choosing between jobs, will it be the job that has better pay or the job that makes you most happy? Here you have to decide, with one I will make more money but is it worth the bitterness that I have to endure or do I prefer to be happier even with a little less pay? More money in my pocket and more stress? It depends on your decision, all of us pass through difficult stages where you don't know what do decide maybe because we might hurt someone. I know that divorce makes you think that you made a bad decision, that you messed up and didn't complete the mission you set out to do, but one must think, "I learned that which I needed to learn." Don't blame yourself over nothing, don't mourn over nothing, at that moment it was the best decision. If everything doesn't turn out like you'd like it to and you don't feel happy and completely accomplished then take it as if you filled a very important space in the other person's life at the most opportune time. You enjoyed everything that you lived up to that moment. Also, if you have stayed married to your ideal companion, why not be even happier making every day a new adventure in your life…whether at dinner time, beginning the day, or going out to eat every now and then, play together, share, dance, give each other quality moments of intimacy, don't become monotonous. Get away from the normal routine because like the song says "love runs out" if it's not nourished like plants without water that wither away, and it does happen even in the best families.

You have a beautiful garden of roses and flowers to take care of. Constantly watering it with clean water, fertilizing the soil, making sure insects don't get to them, trimming them and the sun does the rest. It's the same with our relationship it depends on our determination to do that which we know we need to do! I imagine you're sitting there thinking you're right!!! But be determined right now to do something for yourself and decide that this will be for your own good beginning today. But remember if you have to love your neighbor as yourself, begin to really love yourself and take care of yourself first and you'll see that it will be easier to have love toward everyone else, also, your spouse is your neighbor. Go and save your love, I don't believe that you'll want to start this diet being depressed, it's time!

The true art of love is falling in love over and over again with the same person...

You need good health to give 100% to all the points that we just mentioned.

Harmony in life

Everything in life is based on harmony: Why do we think that everything should be in harmony? It's not about perfectly balancing everything we do simply because we're not perfect. Think about music, every song and its accompaniment: base, piano, guitar, saxophone, percussion and the voices harmonizing a melody that delights the ear and enlightens our soul and spirit. Every instrument is different from the next, they each produce a different sound but all of them fine-tuned together make song, a melody. This is harmony. There are people who can be very good in business but a failure in their marriage, excellent students but horrible at administrating their business, great at love but a failure in their studies and unstable in work…or millionaires and their health at risk, a disaster in their marriage and indecisive. There are doctors that are obese or have diabetes…there are many keys to harmonizing our lives. It doesn't mean that just because someone has a lot of money that they're rich! There are plenty of people that are so poor that they only have money.

They need to harmonize, you must harmonize every part of your life like composing a musical. I like this part because without being perfect we can achieve the inner peace and happiness we're looking for.

Sometimes we have many things that we just don't appreciate. Because we don't conform and are always looking for something more, we begin to choose the instruments that we want; finances, relationship with others, spiritual, mental and physical. Tuning each of these notes cordially harmonizes life which in turn will make us happier and lighten our load…each one of us has the power to make each note better and better until it is perfect. It's just a matter of understanding how we tune and take care of each note. Let's describe each of them just to illustrate a little of what they mean. I'm going to start with health which is the reason for the book.

Health

Without our health we will not be willing or able to do many of the important things in life because one day in our life this machine with stop working properly and the flaws and lamenting begin. As I write this book I'm 49 years old and can read any book without needing glasses. The abusing of our bodies will deteriorate it piece by piece and kids who are born with deficiencies, those deficiencies come in part because of the parents not giving their bodies what they needed both before pregnancy and during. Heritage and genes the cause a lot of time as well and are unpredictable. Some bodies come in to the world prone to illness, for this reason if we teach and help our young ones to take of themselves, eating healthy, they won't suffer as much when they grow up. If our temple doesn't have energy to even get up early or energy to exercise then there is something that we have been doing wrong and it's not functioning at its highest potential, we are wasting away our days. So we'll cover this in more detail in the next paragraph on only health

HEALTH

Having a smoothie of the following greens first thing in the morning is excellent to maintain a longer, healthier life full of energy:

Celery, Asparagus, cucumber, spinach, lettuce, avocado, nopal (cactus), kiwi, green beans, green grapes, green apple, pear, radish, carrot, watercress, mango, banana, strawberry to make it sweet and a more pleasant taste…preferably no sugar added. Leave out banana, strawberry and mango for the diabetic. Every fruit and every vegetable in its season. It's preferable to use all natural for better results, mix it with apple juice or natural organic pear juice or homemade with an extractor.

One or two limes helps to maintain a neutral flavor and it lasts longer. Even then it's better to drink it within 25 minutes of preparing it. It should be consumed while fresh, remember it's liquid salad. It will never do you harm even if you drink it in excess.

If you want to lose weight and feel healthier eliminate carbonated drinks and its derivatives (sodas, sweeteners, dyes, etc. nor drinks that say diet or light). Do you want better results? Don't eat late at night (eat dinner before 5pm) only a cup of natural V10, a salad and you will see the changes and of course consult with your doctor before doing this. The key to this is that it will help to maintain your body alkaline and no sickness can enter an alkaline body. It's rich in antioxidants that purify your organism, cleans your colon, and it's much better for you than a cup of coffee for breakfast. You'll will realize that your body has been asking for it all along.

Every death caused by illness is unnatural (that means that every sickness is caused by our poor eating). There is only one sickness and that's self-intoxication. We think that drinking a cup of coffee, a soda, a pastry or donut is feeding our bodies, but it's putting our bodies in an acidic state and accelerates cancer. You need 32 cups of water to purify your body of one soda pop drank. We are prematurely making ourselves old.

Why do you think pharmacies exist? To sell us what our bodies lack, vitamins that are scarce in us, remedies to calm that with which we have intoxicated ourselves, vitamins that are found in fruits and vegetables because we don't ingest them throughout the whole day. Besides that our body is balanced by PH. Medically it's measured on a scale of 1-14, if your PH is 7 or a little more you will always be healthy alkaline. PH (potential hydrogen)

(1-2 (-3.5-4-5.5)-6--   7   +8+9+10+11+12+13+14)
ACIDIC cancer--------neutral------ALKALINE total health

A body with a -3.5 to -5.5 acidic is where cancer is activated. While a body in alkalinity does not get sick.

And you might ask…

What makes your body alkaline?

The greens that our Creator gave us since Adam and Eve. God said: "…I have given you every herb bearing seed, which is upon the face of all the earth, and every tree, in the which is the fruit of a tree yielding seed; to you it shall be for meat." (Genesis 1:29 KJV)

He didn't say every soda or potato chip, or every fatty, fried food and excess of sweets shall be for meat. If you want to damage your health and live with illness in your old age and grow old faster than normal do the opposite of what God taught centuries ago. Also, the pancreas which produces natural insulin of the body only feeds on greens. Without greens the pancreas dies off slowly of hunger and you turn diabetic and a diabetic is a dead pancreas of which there is no cure.

You don't want to be diabetic right? Eat greens every single day.

Now, fruits should be eaten on an empty stomach preferably in the morning because the intestines are that which digest them and not the stomach, and that's what will purify the colon, and also, it's where fiber does its work.

And we know that the majority of these vegetables are good for our skin, which you can actually use on the skin. The best result will always be from the inside out.

We must exercise every day whether it's walking, bicycling, or walking the dog. There are many ways to exercise. Start with 10-25 min. daily, by doing this we will be more energized and healthy. All doctors recommend exercising regularly.

Also, we can change our metabolism by eating smaller portions every three hours like; an apple, almonds, oat bars, granola, nuts in general, grapes, orange, etc. This will accelerate the metabolism y will cause us to lose weight. Breakfast and lunch should be bigger meals but not dinner. Dinner should be small. You can drink a V10 Natural which in this book I'll show you how to make. You can make special and nutritious smoothies with protein and vitamins. Don't eat fruits at night, fruits only in the morning and afternoon unless they are acidic like pineapple.

DRUBINLIFE

This special formula contains all that your body needs and if any of these ingredients are not good for you, you can leave it out (not because you don't like it but if you are allergic to one of the ingredients) but all of these ingredients are beneficial for your body.

I have selected 11 vegetables and 6 fruits all of which are miraculous and rich in healing properties and properties that will prevent any sickness in your body. Here I we will give you the information of each of the fruits and veggies so that as you eat you can think on the health benefits of what you're partaking. I have done a thorough investigation and here is everything that each of them do. Don't forget to consult your doctor if you have any doubt about this.

Ingredients and measurements of Drubinlife (equivalent to 1 liter)
Important note: Clean each of the thoroughly before using.

1 Celery (1 complete stick of celery), ½ Green Apple, ½ pear, 6 Green Beans, 12 Green Grapes (12-15), Spinach (two handfuls), 1 Kiwi (small, whole with skin), 2 sticks of Watercress, ½ Mango (with the skin but not the seed), 1 Carrot (small), 2 Strawberries (with the green leaf) 1 Lettuce leaf, 1 Banana (just the banana, no peel), Nopal- Cactus Leaf (about ½ the size of your palm), ½ Avocado (without skin or seed), 2 Radishes (with skin and leaves), ½ cucumber (with skin), 1 sprig Asparagus, 2 small spears of Broccoli.

Mix all of it in a blender with apple juice and all the fiber and skins (except the seeds of the apple, avocado, mango and banana peel…) (sometimes I use ½ cup coconut water)

Every morning drink this concentrated juice of Drubinlife (Green Smoothie). The power of greens...now let's analyze the properties so that you know the true benefits that you're putting in your body...

Celery

The benefits of celery to lose weight are based on its properties to cure obesity:

- **Diuretic**: Thanks to the substances that it is composed of like: salt, limonene, asparagine; we can say it increases the elimination of excess liquid, helping not only to lose weight but, also, to control blood pressure.
- **Low contribution of calories**: 100 grams of celery is only 17 calories.
- **Satisfying**: Thanks to its high fiber content, celery keeps your appetite regular.
- **Purifier**: Because of its high soluble fiber count, it's excellent for purifying the intestines, eliminating all types of toxins that are found there.

Besides having the obesity curing properties of celery, this vegetable possesses other virtues like:

- Reduces blood cholesterol
- Betters circulation which in turn benefits the cardiovascular system
- Helps in eliminating uric acid
- Acts as a sedative and tranquilizer
- It's an antioxidant because it contains vitamin C, E and minerals like selenium, copper, magnesium, iron, phosphorus, etc.

As you see, besides helping you to lose weight, it's beneficial to your overall health. Don't doubt it, nature is wise and gives you everything that you need.

Green Beans

French beans, string beans, namely green beans are immature fruits of various Fabaceae species- technically legumes. They are pods that are flattened and elongated whose interior is made up of seeds that vary according to its specie. Even though in the maturing process the walls of the green bean harden through the formation of fibrous tissue, in their immature form they are edible and are consumed as vegetables.

Although some historians affirm that they're of Asian origin, the majority of them originate in America. Precisely, the green bean was one of the foods that was found by the European colonists in the American conquest. The green bean's arrival to Spain took place a few years later with the returning expeditions from the new world, even though then they were only used for their seeds.

From a botanical point of view, French beans belong to the legume or leguminous plant family, specifically to the green bean group. Due to its form of consumption and nutritious properties they are considered vegetables.

Green beans possess a low energetic value, being that they have 30 Kcal/ 100 gm, almost 90% of its weight is water, 4-5% carbohydrates, 2.5% fiber and 2% protein. Its content is found in the micronutrients-vitamins and minerals. Canned green beans do not have the same composition as do the fresh ones. As a result being cooked in autoclaves they absorb water and as a result they have some vitamin loss, the same is true with the traditional way we cook them at home.

We can determine the carotenoid content in fresh green beans is 40% more than cooked green beans and 20% more iron in fresh than cooked, as well. Summarizing, we can say that a 175 gm of green beans carries 30 Kcal, 13% daily value of fiber, at least 17% daily value of iron, 28% of the folic acid requirements, 20%

recommended intake of vitamin A and in turn 5% of B group vitamins.

Properties: Green beans represent a very digestible food, with a diuretic and purifying effect that prevents and betters Hepatic Pathologies.

Rich in vitamins A, B6 and C, in folic acid and fiber, these legumes do not have fats. With these properties, green beans can be part of any weight loss diet.

Calcium, found in green beans, helps in the growth of our children, pregnancy, and menopause and with illnesses such as osteoporosis. Like the rest of legumes, green beans are a fountain of iron and are very recommendable in the diets of those who suffer from anemia. Consuming green beans lowers the level of sugar in the blood stream, therefore diabetics benefit greatly and they also alleviate rheumatic pain.

Spinach:

It's not a coincidence that the feeble Popeye needed a can of spinach every time had to defend Olive from the harassment of Brutus. In fact, the fame that this vegetable gets is deserved, notwithstanding, its nutritious properties are many. Not only does it give you energy and strength, but it's also light and doesn't have a single gram of fat.

The caloric content of spinach is minimal: 100 gm of this vegetable has only 16 calories. It doesn't have cholesterol or fat either, which makes it an indispensable ingredient in any weight loss diet.

Spinach is considered a powerful source of minerals, and is full of iron above all. The amount of these minerals are important. Not only does its absorption vary, but also, this vegetable possesses a large quantity of magnesium, calcium, phosphorus, potassium and sodium. Therefore, they're vital in the diet of our kids and adolescents. The leaves possess an abundance of folic acid, essential to the formation of blood. But, at the same time, they provide an important amount of uric acid and oxalic. Because of this, those who suffer from gout, kidney stones or arthritis should consult their specialist so that they can recommend the adequate amount they should consume.

As for its vitamins, spinach has a lot of beta-carotenes, precursory of vitamin A. They are also rich in vitamin B9, which carries and important anti-carcinogen function. Spinach also has vitamin C, but it loses it when it's cooked. Because of this, when one is lacking vitamins, it's better eat this vegetable in a salad or in the Drubinlife.

Component	Raw Spinach	Boiled Spinach
Lipids (g)	0.35	0.26
Protein (g)	2.86	2.97
Carbohydrates (g)	3.5	3.75
Calcium (mg)	99	136
Iron (milligrams)	2.71	3.57
Magnesium (mg)	79	87
Phosphorus (mg)	49	56
Potassium (mg)	558	466
Sodium (mg)	79	70
Vitamin C (mg)	28.1	0.76
Vitamin E (mg)	1.89	9.8
Vitamin B6 (mg)	0.2	0.955
Cholesterol (mg)	0	0
Fiber (g)	2.7	2.4

Watercress:

Alkalinity
With 65% base salts, watercress is an alkalizing food.

Calories

Watercress has only 23 calories for each 100 grams.

How to choose watercress

It's better to consume this plant really fresh. With time its elements deteriorate and become toxic. If you see that the leaves are withered or yellowed, you should get rid of it. Neither should you eat them if they have flowered or blossomed.

Effects on your organism:

Because of its iodine, sulfur, phosphates, potassium oxalate, other mineral salts and vitamins it's tonic, refreshing, antiscorbutic (prevents scurvy), appetizing, anti-anthelmintic (kills intestinal worms), stimulating and blood tonic. Its action is very notable on infarcts of the liver. Its anti-diabetic properties are notable, as well. It's a diuretic, purifies the stomach, kidneys and bladder.

Its iron content bestows a powerful action on the regeneration of hemoglobin. Its essential sulphureted oils explains its antitussives and its action on the mucus secretion of the respiratory apparatus. Finally, some investigators attribute its restrictive effects on the development of cancer. It strengthens equilibrium, particularly people who are weak, deficient, anorexic, asthenic, anemic, lymphatic, scrofulous, rachitic, undernourished, bronchitic, tuberculosis, and ganglion. All of which are highly benefited by the extraordinary, vitalizing virtues of which this plant has been blessed. Also, it's recommendable for youth who are struggling with adolescence, those with eczema and diabetes, draining the extra sugar through urine.

It can form part of a hypo-caloric regimen designed to combat obesity, as well as in cases of urinary stones, atony of the digestive system, dropsy and as an expectorant for chronic chest cold.

Finally, being that it is an antidote to nicotine, smokers should eat it to fight coughing. Around a 100 grams can be administered daily in juice form mixed with milk or cold broth, being that if it's mixed with hot liquids its curing virtues will evaporate. Therefore, it's a great ingredient for drubinlife.

<u>CARROTS</u>

- Carrots are one of the richest foods in beta-carotene, ideal for the eyes and skin. But also, they're full of many other nutrients and properties, and a great mineralizer.
- Its juice is purifying and alkalizing.
- Carrots stimulate the elimination of waste and help to dissolve gall stones thanks to its beta-carotene content.
- It's ideal for skin problems
- It favors night vision because of its great richness of vitamin A.
- It balances metabolic and digestive problems.
- Carrots are good for getting rid of gas
- In its composition is a high percentage of beta-carotene which is converted to vitamin A if Vitamin A is lacking in the body. At the same time it collaborates in absorbing iron.
- The contribution of potassium in carrots maximizes kidney activity helping to eliminate toxins.
- They offer vitamin C. More than anything through their leaves. You can prepare tasty soup with them, although most carrots are sold without the leaves.
- Their iron content makes them a useful complement in cases of anemia.
- Even though it's found with a lesser quantity, they also offer both vitamins B6 and E.
- Eating an excess of carrots can provoke deposits of carotene below the skin, giving your skin a yellow tone.
- You will benefit from all of these properties simply by consuming 85 grams of carrots per day.

LETTUCE

The curing properties of lettuce are very notable. Comparing its acid-forming elements to its alkalizing elements, lettuce is highly alkaline. It's because of this that it constitutes a powerful neutralizing food against acids which benefits the bad results of having too much acid in the blood and tumors.

It's very useful for rheumatism, arthritis, gout, acidosis, diabetes, cutaneous eruptions, eczema, varicose veins, arteriosclerosis, etc. Because of this it's wise to eat lettuce in abundance every day.

Multi-function Natural Cooking

The little silicon that is has is essential for hair, nails, skin, tooth enamel and all of the cellular tissue walls.

Lettuce isn't a nutritive nor a stimulant, but it's good for irritated nerves and nervousness, to wake up your appetite, to increase the urine flow and for insomnia. The lettuce cortex that has grown to complete maturity contains lactucin which can be used to prepare a magnificent calming meal and is prepared in the following manner:

Add to 1 Liter of water 2 to 3 lettuce stalks cut in little pieces, crushed up in a pan and bring it to a boil until the water is reduced to about half and then pass it through a strainer.

This concoction has magnificent results with affected respiratory pathways especially with colds and bronchitis. The effects will be even better if you add to the concoction the same amount of marshmallow root, flaxseed or any other type of mucilaginous plant, sweetening it with brown sugar or preferably with honey. In this way you will have the soothing effects of broncho-pulminary mucus and an excellent expectorant.

This concoction is also efficient against stomach pain, you'll just want to drink a cup every 3 hours.

Besides this, another way it can be used for abdomen pain is by applying it in the form of an enema. Mix 2 or 3 cups of this concoction with water of plantain, mallow, or flaxseed.

The leaves infused with burned brown sugar is good to combat insomnia and the suppression of urine. Lettuce boiled with a little bit of salt is useful for dyspepsia and to strengthen the stomach, in this case you should eat it in the morning. Prepare a few cooked and chopped up lettuce leaves, drink one cup before going to bed. This is excellent for those who don't sleep well, lack sleep and it will fight asthma attacks and chest colds.

Insomnia

To fight off insomnia one can drink 2 cups of extracted lettuce trunk before going to bed.

The results are very good for menstruation (difficult or painful for women). Besides that, it's a main remedy in the vagotonic crisis, pelvis congestion, for overcrowded hemorrhoids, gallbladder pain and melancholy. In all of these cases, you'll want to boil 60 grams of lettuce in one liter of water and drink three cups a day. And of course, blended up in the Drubinlife every morning will give you even better results.

External Applications of Lettuce

The utilized superficial applications of lettuce is very diverse. In its cooked state it is excellent to calm your nerves, in which it can be used in warm bathes. Lettuce leaves with olive oil applied to the forehead will fight insomnia and should be taken off immediately when the patient has fallen asleep.

Lettuce in the form of a heat compress constitutes a great emollient for inflammation and a great relaxer.

Cooking full grown lettuce stalk, boiled in water, reduced down to half, adding in plantain or mallow gets great results with tooth aches and inflammation in the gums. In these cases you'll want to use it like mouthwash various times during the day.

Lettuce boiled for ten minutes and then applied in the form of a compress with a little bit of olive oil, brings down inflammation of swelling or lumps and takes away the skin redness.

Lettuce juice is magnificent for treating erysipelas and its inflammations. For this you'll apply in compress form to the affected regions. Distilled lettuce water can be used for diseased eyes in the form of eye drops.

Cactus Leaf (Nopal)

The utilization of cactus leaves varies in that it can be consumed in juices, candies, salads and soups to name a few.

Taking advantage of the curing properties of this plant is a millennial practice that has never stopped existing. In the case of cactus leaf in Mexico, it has a special significance for the symbolic role it played in the settlement of the Aztecs at Lake Texcoco, giving way to its empire Tenochtitlan (te- tea, piedra- stone and nochtli- nopal(cactus leaf)). The Aztecs used it for many different medicines: they drank the juice to lower fevers, they used the mucilage (gummy substance) to cure chapped lips, the pulp cured diarrhea, the needles to clean infections. The fruit was used for the excess of bile, the leaves as a warm bandage to alleviate inflammation and the root was used to treat hernias, irritated liver, stomach ulcers and erysipelas. At present it is part of the national shield of Mexico and it still has medicinal uses and various nutritional values.

Nopal(cactus leaf) is a wild plant that survives in desert and cold regions. It doesn't require a lot of water to cultivate, which makes a good source of income for many agricultural farmers who don't rely on necessary resources and live in arid or semi-arid zones. It is said that they play an important ecological role being that they keep deforested land from degrading, in other words they convert unproductive land in to productive land. There exists about 1,600 species and 122 different types of cactus in the cactus family, in which provides nopal. They have fruit which is edible and are known as prickly pear.

Nutrition Properties

Nopal is used as forage but at the same time its soft leaves are commercialized as a vegetable. They can be pickled, cooked in broth and soups, in salads or stews, as a main dish, as snacks, salsas, drinks, deserts, jams, etc. Basically the uses of nopal are never ending for this plant that has such rich properties. Recently, the consumption of nopal has been very popular blended up with other fruit (like in Drubinlife) as a measure to lose weight or for people who suffer from certain illnesses which we'll describe in a minute. The only problem with nopal is that many people find the mucilage a little unpleasant, being that it stays in the smoothie. Cactus powder or dehydrated cactus has offered a solution for this inconvenience. To avoid the mucilage of nopal you can freeze it or strain it. Also, it is recommended to add to the juice garlic, baking soda, tomato skin, corn leaf, lemon juice, ash or volcanic rock.

Nutritional Properties

With respect to the nutritional value of nopal, it can be said that in 1 cup of raw nopal (approximately 86 grams) there are 2.9 g. of carbohydrates, 1.1 g. of protein and only Kcal. But its main attraction is that it has a good quantity of dietetic fiber (soluble and insoluble): 2 g. of fiber per cup. It has a proportion of 30:70 soluble fiber to insoluble. Insoluble fiber can prevent and alleviate constipation and hemorrhoids while at the same time prevent the appearance of colon cancer. Soluble fiber has been used many times for those suffering with digestive issues but because its presence in the digestive tract slows down the absorption of nutrients it makes it so that they don't pass to the bloodstream as fast. Nopal is also a great source of calcium, being that in 100 g. of nopal there is approximately 80 mg of calcium.

Medicinal Properties

It has been demonstrated in many studies, especially those done in Mexico, which the medicinal properties of nopal help to control illness. This doesn't mean it's used to heal.

Obesity. It has become very popular in all diets to drink cactus juice with orange or some other fruit. This is because of the quantity of fiber that this plant has. It helps to slow down the time it takes to absorb nutrients and for them to enter the blood and therefore making is elimination easier. Also, the soluble fiber that is has creates a sensation of fullness, lowering the level of hunger that one has and helps for good digestion. At the same time, the vegetable proteins promote mobilization of liquids in the blood stream reducing cellulitis and water retention.

Diabetes and hyperglycemia. Also, it is said that it helps those individuals who suffer with diabetes. Nopal increases the levels and the sensibility of insulin, stabilizing and regulating blood sugar level. It has been proven scientifically the hyperglycemic power of nopal. This means that is an effective treatment for the prevention of diabetes. They have carried out investigations at the National Polytechnic Institute where it is documented that nopal reduces glucose concentrations in the blood. In these studies it has been shown that ingesting nopal before every meal during 10 days reduces body weight along with glucose concentrations, cholesterol and triglycerides in the blood. This has only been seen in people who are resistant to insulin, in other words, in patients that have type 2 diabetes (they don't produce insulin). Note: Nopal doesn't substitute insulin shots.

Cholesterol. In people with high cholesterol, it has been shown that the consumption of nopal helps to eliminate it. The amino acids, fiber and niacin content in nopal prevents the excess of sugar in the blood which converts to fat. While at the same time it metabolizes the fat and fatty acids therefore reducing cholesterol. The LDL (low-density lipoprotein) content in nopal is believed to be the main cause that cholesterol is expulsed from the body, being that the LDL acts on the same level as the liver removing and getting rid of excess cholesterol in the body. At the same time, it has been observed that this quantity of LDL doesn't affect HDL (high density lipoprotein) or "good" cholesterol. Nopal has a sufficient amount of amino acids and fiber; including antioxidants vitamin C and A, which prevent the possibility of damaging blood vessels and also the formation of plaque. For this same reason it is a powerful preventative in relation to atherosclerosis.

Antibiotic property. Nopal has natural antibiotics. This property is related to CAM (crassulacean acid metabolism) of plants, which in cactus it inhibits or suspends the growth of various species of bacteria. With that being said, the consumption of nopal or the application of cactus leaf as a bandage have beneficial effects on wounds and skin infections.

Cancer. In an experiment done with rats with cancerous tumors, watery extracts of Opuntia maxim (substance that is found in nopal) was administered and they found that it prolonged the latency period of said malignant tumors

It didn't cure the cancer but it detained it. They don't know the cause yet but they are doing various studies with respect to this.

Gastrointestinal and digestive disorders. Finally, it is known that vegetable fibers and mucilage control excess gastric acids and protect gastrointestinal mucus preventing gastric ulcers and all types of affections. Nopal contains vitamins A, B complete, C, minerals: calcium, magnesium, sodium, potassium, iron, and fiber in lignin, cellulose, hemicellulose, pectin, and mucilage; all that with 17 amino acids help to eliminate toxins. Environmental toxins contributed by alcohol and cigarette smoke that inhibit the immune system are eliminated by nopal. It will also clean the colon since it contains dietary fibers both soluble and insoluble. The insoluble dietary fibers absorb water and accelerate the time it takes for food to pass through the digestive tract and contribute to regulate intestinal movement. Besides that, the presence of insoluble fiber in the colon dilutes concentrated carcinogens that could be present. And it's a main ingredient in Drubinlife.

AVOCADO:

Avocado is a fruit which helps to better the life of those who consume it being that it has the majority of required elements for a healthy diet, preventing illnesses and in some cases helping to heal them. We know that avocado, besides being excellent in salads and some of our favorite dishes, helps in fortifying our abdominal muscles collaborating in reducing the "pop belly" and functions as a cardiac protector. It contains minerals, vitamins, acids and amino acids. More than anything, it's actually a curing agent for various sicknesses not only for women but also men. Besides the pulp containing a large quantity of mono-unsaturated fatty acids which are very appropriate to control cholesterol and triglycerides, it contains vitamins from the B group. It has a protecting effect on the cardiac muscle, which it is suggested that that you consume at least 2 avocados per week.

It is not enough to know that this food possesses large quantities of vitamin E which is favorable for the skin, hair, and nails for the women who are always looking for ways to look beautiful, but also it acts as a protection from cardiac illnesses. This type of food has always been used because of its curing properties. It has its properties, but we must understand that it doesn't work like medicine does immediately. Besides consuming it, it's an excellent ally of beauty. It can be applicated in diverse treatments for your hair and skin. The fruit that have a greater quantity of vitamin E are: kiwi, nectarine, grapes and peaches. But in all reality there are thousands of recipes of different cultures in which you can apply avocado, like guacamole, chicken salad, sushi and others. What would you put it in? It has dermatological virtues that are the base of numerous cosmetic products: creams, soaps, emulsions, being that its pulp contributes to the regeneration of tissue.

Benefits of Avocado

1- It's useful in fighting against cholesterol and the prevention of arteriosclerosis.
2- It stimulates collagen formation. Because of this, it helps combat the aging of skin.
3- It helps with problems like eczema, dermatitis and pimples.
4- Its smoothing properties from avocado seed (avocado oil) are used in the cosmetic industry to elaborate products for the skin and hair.
5- Because of its vitamin D, it helps in the absorption of calcium and phosphorus.
6- It delays the aging process because of it vitamin E content.
7- It helps people with diabetes being that is equalizes sugar in the blood stream.
8- Helps with dry skin.
9- Helps with physical effort (as with athletes)
10- It's great for pregnant women.

Ally of the heart? Avocado has oleic acid, a type of fat that helps to reduce cholesterol levels. Its consumption is recommended in diets to control cholesterol but because of its elevated caloric contribution one shouldn't abuse the ingestion thereof. According to a new study, avocado has almost double the vitamin E that it was thought to have which is very beneficial being that this vitamin is known for delaying the aging process and protecting against cardiac illnesses and common types of cancer.

Used as a conditioner for hair, avocado helps to restructure hair and make it shine, moisturizing and reviving it. One of way of applying it is simply making a puree chopping up the pulp preferably when it has ripened. Apply it to your hair, leave it for about 20 minutes so that the fatty acids absorb in and then wash out. You will notice the difference immediately. You can add to it a teaspoon of pure olive oil if you prefer even better results. In place of using the pulp of avocado you can use just avocado oil in the same way.

Skin Moisturizer

Avocado contributes many benefits for your skin, especially in lifeless looking skin, dry, mixed and aging skin. You can make a mask of avocado puree and a table spoon of honey for you face. Before you go to bed, leave it on for about 30 minutes and then remove it. Another option is apply avocado oil directly to your skin. Avocado is a pharmaceutical veggie, its infused leaves are good for the gall bladder and are anti-flatuants, diuretics, and anti-rheumatic. It alleviates bronchitis, snoring and menstrual cramps. As a local application it has certain anti-inflammatory properties and helps to calm head-aches. The oil that comes from the pulp is used to give massages for gout and rheumatoid or as a lotion to fight dandruff or loss of hair. The specialist also referred to antioxidants, "A new study has found that beans are also an important part of our diet, "Especially red or colored because they have more antioxidant elements. Raspberries, strawberries, pink fish, salmon, sardines, nuts, corn, oranges, broccoli, peppers, apples, olives, onions, artichokes. And these are very important as we to fight against and neutralize free radicals that are common in our daily lives as well as to strengthen our own defenses. Pollution, UV rays and alcohol decreases the body's ability to fight free radicals, which contributes to premature aging and disease. Foods containing vitamin C and E, beta-carotene and the mineral selenium are powerful antioxidants. Avocado also provides smoothness and a pleasant flavor to Drubinlife.

RADISH:

The benefits of raphanus sativus (radishes) are one of those vegetables that despite its carbohydrate content, they are still low in calories and offer a large supply of water. And on the other side, it offers a good amount of fiber, ideal for the digestive system and also to feel full.

In addition to this content, radish also has vitamin C, perfect for teeth, bones and it's valuable for its antioxidant action, as in folate, great for the gestation of red and white blood cells. It is worth adding that radish is packed with minerals.

Calcium is one that is present in radishes, though, sources of calcium of plant origin are generally not as good as that from animals. Radishes also have potassium, ideal for the central nervous system, iodine and magnesium in good proportions and also sulfur, a very good antioxidant.

RADISH: A FOOD WITH MANY THERAPEUTIC PROPERTIES

Although less nutritious than other roots like carrots or beets, radish and especially black radish occupies a prominent place among the foods considered therapeutic recognized for its ability to promote drainage of the liver and gallbladder, stimulate bile production, eliminate the organism's waste and toxins, regulate the functions of the colon or disorder. Digestive addition to fever, intestinal infections, ulcers, cold, rheumatism and gout, to name a few ailments. In addition, several of its active principles which it shares with other members of brassica or cruciferous family, confer important antimicrobial, antioxidant, expectorant, diuretic and immunostimulant properties, also, cleansing and anti-cancer.

Numerous studies conducted in recent years give this member of the brassicaceae family in which it was formerly called cruciferae - an important therapeutic value and it's recognized for its medicinal properties which other foods are don't have therefore they are "highly regarded". As an example, let's say that the botany brassica family comprising over 380 genera and some 3,000 vegetables species comprise the top of the list of anti-cancer vegetables. And is that the glucosinolates, isothiocyanates (including sulforaphane), indoles and other phytochemicals. In addition to the vitamins, minerals and fiber content of broccoli, brussels sprouts, cabbage, red cabbage, cauliflower, and turnips, radish's become essential to maintain health due to their anticancer, antimicrobial, antioxidant, diuretic, cleansing, anti-inflammatory, hepatoprotective, immunostimulant, choleretic, cholagogue, digestive and expectorant properties.

Ancient Remedy

As we said radish belongs to the large family of the Brassicaceae and receives the scientific name Raphanus sativus. It is an edible plant, thick, fleshy root, varies greatly in shape and size and whose skin may be red, pink, white, brown or dark-stained different colors. As for variety the general Raphanus comprises eight different but the most common are Chinese, Japanese or daikon radish (which is cylindrical, elongated, white in color and a smooth taste); radishes (spherical, oval or cylindrical, small, red skin and white, pink or purple skin) and the black radish is cylindrical and rounded, with black skin which is very difficult to digest but whose flesh is white and digestive. And since this is the most commonly used variety of radish for medicinal purposes due to its incontestable therapeutic properties, we will center the text in this. But first it is worth noting that although there is no conclusive data still, it seems that the origin of radish is located in Asia, specifically in China, several thousand years before our era and from there we get that horseradish preparations were prescribed for the treatment of diarrhea, fevers, digestive disorders, intestinal infections, ulcers or flatulence. It is also on record that this vegetable known in ancient

Egypt on some hieroglyphics dating 2700 years before Christ contained references to therapeutic use and cosmetic and also part of the menu of builders of the famous pyramid of Cheops. It was also appreciated by Greeks and the Romans who introduced the cultivation of radish in Spain and spread throughout Europe.

Rich in Potassium

The radish is a root vegetable with high water content. In fact, about 95% of its weight is water, but also, it contains vitamins, minerals and phytochemicals that make it interesting. Although from a nutritional standpoint, it contains less than other members of its family. Thus, the radish is rich in vitamin C and folate (vitamin B). Let us recall that vitamin C is a recognized antioxidant, which is capable of preventing the occurrence of numerous ailments, besides that, it intervenes in the formation of collagen, bones, teeth and red blood cells and enhances the absorption of iron from food and resistance to infection. As for folate, it is involved in the synthesis of genetic material and the formation of antibodies as well as collaborating in the production of both red and white blood cells. With respect to mineral content, it highlights its richness in potassium (needed for the generation and transmission of nerve impulses and normal muscle activity also to intervene in the balance of sodium-potassium cell pump) and their significant amounts of iodine (essential for the proper functioning thyroid regulates metabolism and is involved in growth processes). Also found in it is a certain dose of calcium, phosphorus, iron and magnesium in addition to sulfur (which gives it its spicy flavor). It also contains amino acids (in discrete ratios) and fiber, among other properties which prevent or improve constipation, helps reduce cholesterol levels in blood (decreases intestinal absorption of this lipid) and promotes proper blood sugar control in diabetics. Also contains organic sulfur compounds as the rafanol (of colagog properties, choleretic and antibiotic) and rafanina (lead sulfide compound of black radish that confer antibiotic, antiviral and immuno-stimulants).

But if anything stands out about radishes, especially the black and the brassica, it's safe to say their richness in a number of phytochemicals with proven efficacy for maintaining good health known as glucosinolates and isothiocyanates indoles. The first are the spicy flavorings that are recognized as anticancer properties and the ability to remove harmful or undesirable microbial organisms. The more chew up radish these glucosinolates release other interesting compounds such as isothiocyanates (this root contains allyl isothiocyanate) which is considered to be an effective chemopreventive agent (like sulforaphane, which we'll get more information about later on) or like indoles (radish indometilglucosinolate) favoring detoxification of the organism and may also play a role in preventing breast cancer and ovarian cancer, of which they are doing studies. Well, these elements gives the radish and especially the black radish, for being the most rich of radishes in these therapeutic substances, of which we will continue to analyze.

HEPATOPROTECTOR, BLOOD CLEANER, DIGESTIVE, and ANTICARCINEGEN . . .

If you look on the Internet, or any other source of information data about radish and/or its black variety, of which we speak, we will soon conclude that this vegetable is especially appreciated from the therapeutic point of view for their ability to drain and purify the liver and gallbladder. Thus it is contrasted, for example, that black radish isothiocyanates stimulate contraction of the gallbladder, bile production and emptying of said gland. Following ingestion this result favors the drainage of accumulated debris in both gallbladder and the liver (and by extension removes wastes and toxins accumulated in the body) and helps prevent stone formation. And as you know a good gallbladder favors liver function because, among other things, it "saves" it work. Therefore it is considered that radish is a hepatoprotective and very suitable food in cases of Hepatobiliary deficiencies, digestive disorders linked to an overload liver, biliary secretion disorders, migraines of hepatic origin, etc. But besides being an excellent drainer and liver protector, radish is appreciated for being a diuretic and cleanser. Its high water composition (95% of its weight) and its richness in potassium and some other of its components make the radish a more than appreciated vegetable diuretic favoring increased urination and thereby the removal of toxic substances or waste and expulsion more fast and effective of fluid retained in the body resulting beneficial for those who suffer with hypertension, retain liquids or oliguria. Moreover, as already mentioned, it contributes to both prevent stone formation (liver, bile, kidney, etc.) as to eliminate and expel them if they already exist. But also have found that promotes blood purification, cleaning intestinal and gastric mucosa, removing potentially harmful substances when they accumulate as uric acid, urea, cholesterol, etc. Being that the radish is considered one of the most useful foods for the liver then it can also be considered one of the most beneficial for the digestive system. We say this because in addition to wetting the appetite, it stimulates production of gastric juice, increases or facilitates natural bowel movements, regulates functions of the colon, relieves chronic constipation and bloating and acts as a mild laxative with its fiber content. It also maintains the intestinal flora in a healthy state which, in addition to combating diarrhea and intestinal infections, prevents many infectious diseases. We must also say that it does not contain fat thus it's considered a good partner to stay thin or to integrate into a diet. . . .

Cardio Protective

The increased volume of urine which is expelled by consuming this vegetable helps lower blood pressure and increase diuresis in the body eliminating substances that could lead to cardiovascular complications. Furthermore, the fiber contained in it decreases intestinal cholesterol absorption. Moreover, the potassium and other substances it contains are essential for good blood circulation. Also, its glucosinolate and isothiocyanates are recognized as potent antioxidants action against free radicals which also contributes to reduce cardiovascular and cerebrovascular risk. For these reasons, radish is considered a food with cardio protective activity. . . . immunostimulant. Because of its antioxidant content, radish is considered a food that acts as an immunostimulatory against potentially injurious free radicals. Besides, their isothiocyanates help enzymes to detoxify the body -first line of defense of the organism against sicknesses- it neutralizes the harmful substances that enter it through different routes (diet, pollution, etc.). Thus it is considered to contribute to preventing the development of numerous degenerative conditions helping to prevent cell damage. It's also considered a potent antimicrobial (thanks to a substance called diphenyl peroxide glyoxal) and it is known that its active principles neutralize pathogenic bacteria, especially, virus and fungi-which are housed in the lining of the kidney, bladder, urinary tract, stomach and respiratory tract. Hence, especially in autumn and winter, our grandmothers and other medical traditions such as the Chinese recommend drinking radish juice to prevent or alleviate symptoms such as respiratory ailments like colds, flu, bronchitis, etc.

Anti-carcinogenic

As mentioned earlier in this text brassicas lead the list of considered plants thanks to their anticancer richness and isothiocyanates and in this respect the most emphasized is sulforaphane – a cancer fighting agent not only for their ability to modulate the aforementioned detoxification enzymes of the body but also because they have anti-inflammatory activity, antibacterial and antiviral in addition to inducing selective apoptosis of cancer cells, they inhibit the formation of new blood vessels that can feed the tumor and avoid the dividing of the cancer cell. Radish also contains these interesting substances in important proportions, according to the latest research, it may be useful to prevent cancers of different tissues including lung, mammary gland, ovaries, esophagus, liver, gallbladder, pancreas, bladder, prostate, small intestine or colon, to name a few.

But also, radish is good for:

-   It is rich in folate so it's considered suitable for pregnant women and that a deficiency of these vitamins during the first weeks of pregnancy can cause defects such as anencephaly and spinal bifida in the baby.
-   Promotes expectoration in cases of respiratory disease.
-   Being an antibacterial and promotes blood purification and helps improve conditions such as acne.
-   Helps you lose weight because it favors the elimination of liquids, waste substances and accumulated fats.
-   The consumption of black radish juice and artichoke has a regulatory effect metabolism lipid in the liver and helps maintain adequate levels of cholesterol and triglycerides.
-   For its wealth of vitamins and minerals which help in cases of anemia.
-   Has relaxing properties and facilitates sleep.
-   Used topically it's effective as a reliever of osteo inflammation.
-   For its antiseptic and antimicrobial capacity which helps improve the state of the skin in cases of eczema, wounds, lacerations, burns, etc. (washing injuries with juice or using a poultice). In short, an excellent alternative natural way to maintain health and help the body prevent numerous ailments.

CHOOSING AND PRESERVING THEM

Radish is another one of those seasonal products that, fortunately, we have year round. And it's common that people only use the root but there are some people who use their leaves as if they were spinach or to make infusions. Otherwise it is customary to consume it raw, especially by those who appreciate the spicy flavors. You can form part of a salad but also, you can boil, fry, blend with other vegetables, use it for making sauces, etc. If you want to remove the spiciness simply peel the radish. It is the skin that contains most of the substances that give it that quality.

Of course, when choosing, choose the medium sized pieces, fleshy, firm, brightly colored, smooth, seamless and whole skin. And if they still have their leaves they must be intense green because this guarantees its freshness.

Moreover, do not wash until ready to consume. If you want store them just remove the green parts and save the radishes in the refrigerator in perforated plastic bags. If you do it like this its qualities will remain virtually unchanged during at least one week.

We close by mentioning that toxic effects are not known resulting from excessive consumption of radish but it is known that you should not eat it raw if you suffer from gastritis or gastro duodenal ulcers. It can also cause flatulence because it contains fiber and sulfur compounds, especially among those who have trouble digesting vegetables. In such cases it should be consumed in moderation and preferably boiled.

Properties

Radish, especially black, is:

- Anti anemic.
- Anti carcinogen.
- Anti scorbutic.
- Anti spasmodic.
- Anti-inflammatory.
- Antimicrobial.
- Antioxidant.
- Antiseptic.
- Soothing.
- Carminative.
- Colagogo.
- Choler etic.
- Detoxifying.
- Digestive.

- Diuretic.
- Expectorant.
- Hepatoprotector.
- Immune.
- Laxative.
- Relaxing.
- Rubefacient (topical use).
- Sedative.
- Vitamin.

Indications

- Acne.
- Asthma.
- Bronchitis.
- Kidney stones.
- Cancer.
- Cystitis.
- Cholecystitis.
- Colitis with constipation.
- Diarrheal colitis.
- Slow digestion.
- Dyspepsia hypo secretors.
- Hepatobiliary dyskinesia.
- Eczema (topical use).
- Emphysema.
- Scurvy.
- Constipation.
- Pharyngitis.
- Drop.
- Flu.
- Hepatitis.
- Hypertension.
- Hyperuricemia.
- Jaundice.
- Loss of appetite.

- Intestinal infections.
- Inflammation of the bladder.
- Musculoskeletal inflammations (topical use).
- Skin injuries.
- Bloating.
- Myalgia (topical use).
- Migraines of hepatic origin.
- Oliguria.
- Biliary and hepatic pathologies.
- Problems of intestinal transit.
- Colds.
- Fluid retention.
- Rheumatism.
- Sinusitis.
- Cough irritant.
- Elevated transaminases.
- Sleep disorders.
- Urolithiasis.

CUCUMBER

Cucumber is a food easy to digest when used naturally and can even be used with the skin when it is fresh. It must be eaten without vinegar and preferably unsalted, as it is these things that make cucumber an indigestible food. It is proven that cucumber, used naturally, is not only an easily digestible food but also refreshing and recommended to neutralize excessive acidity in cases of diabetes, gout, arthritic, etc. Although it's considered to be a very good food for the summer being that it's refreshing, it is recommended to be consumed in any season as it helps blood circulation and also has purifying effects in the intestines.

The cucumber mask is great to provide softness to the skin, remove stains and wrinkles. The case of famous beauties, like the French Ninon de Lencios, who used cucumber juice to rejuvenate her skin, and teaches us to prepare cumber oil to serve these same purposes.

It is prepared as follows: Peel and cut ¼ kilo cucumbers and put in 1 ½ liters of warm (not boiling) olive oil and then, after cooling, it is then passed through a sieve and is ready for use.

Pickled cucumbers are unhealthy and should not be used for beauty purposes.

Healthy Properties of Cucumber

This fruit, commonly considered a vegetable, has a modest concentration of vitamin C. One hundred grams of cucumber provides about 10% of the recommended daily intake- 60 mg / day. Vitamin C is involved in suppressing nitrosamine whose carcinogenicity has been demonstrated. Vitamin C may also protect against various cancers and strengthens the immune system.

Cucumber contains no fat and is low in calories and cholesterol. Of the cancer inhibitory substances found in cucumber are phytochemicals such as phytosterols and terpenes. Some dietitians of old, present the cucumber as a difficult food to digest, and this is true in some ways, although in reality it is because people do not know how to prepare it.

Cucumber should be eaten all natural, only after washed good and pealed. The alternative is to put lemon or yogurt but little or no salt.

There is a disease called toxoplasmosis which can only cured with cucumber. What doctors in the United States recommend consists of eating only raw cucumber for 40 days; which produces a deep detoxification of the body.

Cucumber is widely used in medicine, for its emollient, soothing and refreshing and above all its alkalizing qualities. Cucumber is good in hot weather, especially in summer, thanks to its enormous water content. Good for thirst and for bowel action, it cools the blood and has a purifying effect on intestines. They are also highly recommended, when there is a tendency to necrosis, and in all cases where it is necessary to neutralize excess acidity, as in diabetes, gout, obesity, arthritis, etc.

Laxative

Because of its laxative properties it is advisable in constipation, but it must be chewed. Cucumber salad with lemon juice and olive oil, before meals, is a good remedy for stomach pains and dyspepsia. Its juice is good for inflammation of the digestive tract and the bladder. It's also of great importance to secretions and is magnificent in febrile states, and for blood, brain and nerves. Cucumber juice with honey, is excellent for sicknesses of the throat, like hoarseness, inflammation, angina, etc., for which it's to be taken by tablespoons, depending on how serious it is. Finally, the seeds enjoy diuretic properties.

External Use of Cucumber

Cucumber pulp marinated in alcohol and then distilled "cucumber essence" is used to prepare an ointment for external applications to freshen and soften dry skin. This ointment can also be made with only juice, in which case it will act also as a coolant. The juice is excellent for skin rashes, swelling, etc., because of this it is used in lotions or washes.

It is also great to give softness, remove spots and freckles, make wrinkles disappear and rejuvenate the skin. Against diseases of the throat, cucumber pulp applied as poultice can be used several times a day. The seed emulsion is used against hemorrhoids, rashes, abscesses, and other skin rashes.

Cucumber is a vegetable low in calories due to its reduced carbohydrate content, as compared to other vegetables, and its high water content.

It provides fiber, small amounts of vitamin C, small amounts of vitamin A and vitamin E, and even smaller proportions of vitamin B such as folate, B1, B2 and B3. Found in its skin are small amounts of beta-carotene, but once peeled its content is reduced to almost zero.

Vitamin A is essential for vision, good skin, hair, mucous membranes, bones and for the proper functioning of the immune system.

Folates are involved in the production of red and white blood cells, in the synthesis of genetic material and the formation of antibodies in the immune system.

Vitamin E is involved in the stability of blood cells and fertility. Like vitamin C, it has antioxidant action, and also intervenes in the formation of collagen, red blood cells, bones and teeth; it promotes iron absorption and increases resistance against infections.

Cucumber is not considered a mineral rich vegetable but is abundant in potassium and to a lesser extent has phosphorus and magnesium.

Potassium is a mineral needed for the generation and transmission of nerve impulses and normal muscle activity. Plus, it intervenes with water balance inside and outside the cell.

Phosphorus is involved in the formation of bones and teeth, as well as magnesium. The latter also has to do with bowel operation, it enhances immunity and has a mild laxative effect.

In the composition of cucumber is a small proportion of beta-sisterol; a compound with anti-inflammatory activity and is hypoglycemic, which participates in immune system response.

ESPARAGUS

Within home remedies for weight loss, asparagus is one of the excellent options that you should take into account when to starting a weight loss diet. This way, you will achieve good form while taking in an excellent vegetable like this. But, as you already know, if you don't put forth the effort you will not achieve your goals. Asparagus is good but it doesn't do miracles by itself.

One of the main reasons why asparagus is good for weight loss is its low caloric intake. Only 18 calories per 100 grams of asparagus. It also has very few carbohydrates and total absence of fat, an ideal food to incorporate in any type of diet.

In turn, asparagus is a diuretic. This is great to know when getting ready to start a diet. Why? Because it cleanses your body of toxins and helps expel retained fluids. Bear in mind that, like all diuretic plants, it is not recommended for those with problems kidney.

SLIMMING DOWN PROPERTIES OF ASPARAGUS

Asparagus to lose weight

One of the best vegetables that you can use to lose weight is asparagus. But it must be clear that by itself it is not a miracle worker and must be accompanied by a good diet and exercise. Anyway, it will help you lose weight because of its diuretic capacity and its low amount of calories, therefore it becomes perfect to consume daily.

Data on students of the miraculous properties of asparagus "News on cancer" in 1979 spoke of a man who was diagnosed with incurable lung cancer on 5 March 1971. On April 5 he started asparagus therapy, and X-rays in August showed that the cancer was gone and the data listed several other cases.

Canned asparagus can be just as good as fresh asparagus. You just have to choose the ones that have the least possible number of pesticides and preservatives. Fresh ones can be cooked, crushed up in a blender and even dissolved in a little water to drink and it's also a main ingredient of "Drubinlife". Four tablespoons in the morning and four in the night is ideal, but the dose can be increased if desired.

Asparagus have a protein called histores, which activates the control of cell growth. They are also rich in folic acid, vitamin C, thiamine, vitamin B6, potassium and micronutrients

They have no fat or cholesterol and are very low in calories. Asparagus strengthens blood vessels, tone the body and acts against all types of cancer.

BROCCOLI

Broccoli kills the bacteria responsible for many stomach cancers.

Recent studies published in England by the Institute of Food Research in the UK shows that relatively low amounts of cruciferous vegetables in the diet (broccoli, cauliflower, cabbage), a few servings per week, can reduce the risk of prostate cancer and the risk of cancer becoming more aggressive. This anticancer activity also fights against breast, lung and colon cancer.

According to this study broccoli works by activating genes that prevent development of tumors and other genes that promote the expansion of the tumor. Crucifers such as broccoli and cauliflower contain indole-3-carbinol and sulforaphane which substances have antioxidant and anticancer effects.

Broccoli is also recommended in cases of fibromyalgia and lesions caused by human papillomavirus.

On the other hand, a team of scientists from the University of Warwick, in England have concluded that eating broccoli can reverse the cardiovascular damage caused by diabetes. Warwick scientists found that a component of this plant called active sulforane, a protein in the body called 'nrf2', protects cells and tissues through its antioxidant enzymes. Thus, the enzymes protect blood vessels and greatly reduce the molecules causing cardiovascular damage, which decreases the risk of ailments. In fact, decreased risk of heart attacks and strokes had already been related to the properties of broccoli.

Research conducted at the Roswell Park Cancer Institute showed that broccoli and other cruciferous vegetables like cabbage, cauliflower or Brussel sprouts could help smokers prevent lung cancer but its beneficial effects are higher in ex-smokers. The researchers divided their findings into four subtypes of lung cancer and found that the biggest risk reduction was between small cell carcinoma patients and squamous cells. These two subtypes are associated with more intense smoking.

When you want to detoxify your body, many naturopaths recommend fasting all day just eating broccoli and drinking water and this will clean the body and eliminates toxins. (only for 24 hours when your health will allow, remember consult your physician)

GREEN APPLE

What are the properties of green apples?

Green apples are useful for the wellbeing of your health and it is an important highlight its good taste, so not only are you improving your body when you consume them, but you can also enjoy the refreshing taste.

Green apples are mostly composed of pectin, amino acids, acids, sugars, catechins, quercetin, sorbitol, fiber, calcium, iron, magnesium, nitrogen, phosphorus and potassium, among other things.

This fruit has medicinal properties both in relation to internal and external use. On the level of internal ailments, green apples are an anti-inflammatory of the digestive system, an antacid, anti-diarrheal and a mild laxative; they're a diuretic and cleansing, anticatarral in bronchi or cough cases; anti-cholesterol; hypotensive- reduces blood pressure; a sedative, febrifuge, reduces fevers; antismoking, maintaining a diet with apples helps one to leave the vice of tobacco; and they're anti-carcinogenic.

As for external use, green apples relieve muscle pain, cramps; cider vinegar (apple-derived) is used to remove foot fungus. This type of vinegar is also good for the ear; and prevents odor in the armpits and other properties.

So remember that you'll be doing your body a favor when eating green apples as this will help prevent and improve several diseases. And keep in mind that if you don't like taste of apples you can still use them to relieve some external ailments of your body.

GREEN GRAPES

Subtitles
Antioxidants and Free Radicals
Rich in Fiber
Properties

The health benefits of grapes are derived as much from its nutritious components as a number of other substances, whose properties were the topic of study in recent investigations.

It was about the abundant compounds of sorbitol found in grapes which is responsible for color and flavor. Others such as anthocyanin, tannins and flavonoids, all having a powerful antioxidant action. The anthocyanin is responsible for the color pigments in black and red grapes and is absent in the white varieties. Tannins give the feeling of astringency to green grapes. And with flavonoids, resveratrol is the most recognized.

This is found mainly in the skin of the black and red grapes and has antifungal properties. That is it prevents fungal growth on grapes. Recent scientific studies have shown its effectiveness to inhibit or block tumor growth, therefore the regular consumption of grapes is recommended in cases of cancer and if there are risk factors of cancer.

Antioxidants and Free Radicals

All compounds of grapes have antioxidant capacities. During the processes which takes place in cells there are substances generated which are harmful to the body. These are called free radicals and are directly related to the development of diseases such as cardiovascular, degenerative, cancer and the process of aging itself.

Recent studies show that antioxidants contribute in blocking the formation of these substances. Flavonoids and specifically resveratrol, have the following benefits with regards to circulation in the arteries: vasodilation, which increases the blood flow; reduced platelet aggregation (blood circulates better thereby reducing the risk of forming blood clots) and inhibition of oxidation of the cholesterol LDL-c which triggers its deposits in the arteries and leads to atherosclerosis.

In essence, we can be sure that grapes and (grape juice) are foods that promote good health of the arteries and heart. Added to the benefits of its antioxidant richness is the contribution of the minerals potassium and magnesium, which are involved in the contracting of muscles and the heart.

However, its consumption should be taken into special account for people with kidney failure who require special potassium controlled diets. However, those who take diuretics which remove potassium and people with bulimia, which have self-induced vomiting episodes, have large losses of this mineral and it suits them well to consume these fruits.

Rich in Fiber

Because of their fiber content grapes are a mild laxative. In cases of constipation, it is recommended to consume grapes unpeeled and with seeds, since that is where the substances are found that promote intestinal motility and help regulate its operation.

For those who suffer from a sensitive stomach, it is more convenient to consume grape juice or wine. Because of the richness in sugars, people with diabetes and overweight may eat them but must control the amount.

Moderate amounts of folic acid or folate, an essential vitamin in the processes of cell division and multiplication which takes place in the early months of pregnancy, makes the consumption of grapes a great food for pregnant women to prevent spine bifida and alteration in the development of the nerve system (neural tube) of the fetus.

Due to its special composition, these fruits have a diuretic effect beneficial for hyperuricemia or gout and kidney stones (promotes the excretion of uric acid and its salts), hypertension or other diseases associated with fluid retention.

Oxalic acid contained in black grapes can form salts with certain minerals such as calcium to form calcium oxalate. So consumption has to be taken into account if one is suffering kidney stones because it might aggravate the situation.

Polyphenols and tannins, substances abundant in red varieties of grapes, can trigger migraines in susceptible people.

Properties

Grapes contain organic acids such as tartaric, malic, and also tannin; they are abundant in minerals also, with phosphoric acids, iodine and arsenic. Grapes are rich in vitamins, although poor in vitamin C. They lack fats, so the protein rate is very low.

The composition of grape juice is very similar to breast milk, which that alone indicates all its virtues.

Its high level of sugars (glucose and laevulose) makes it easy to digest, since they are naturally absorbed unlike industrial sugars, in which the liver must work harder to process it. Grapes have plenty of calories, so they are suitable for a normal diet. Grapes are a good laxative and anti-diarrheal, and are used for kidney ailments. The application of consuming grapes is used to combat obesity. Grapes also detoxify the body and are useful for fevers and stomatitis. Grapes rejuvenate the skin and cure pimples. Regarding raisins, one must understand that yes they are grapes but you shouldn't abuse the consumption of them, since you are obligated to eat them with wrinkled skin. Raisins are even more of a laxative than grapes, taken in small amounts. When fresh grapes are missing raisins can replace almost all of its advantages.

KIWI:

KIWI, AUTHENTIC HEALTH TREASURE

Kiwi contains minerals, protects the heart and skin, strengthens the immune system, improves digestion, prevents cancer and high cholesterol and retards cellular aging.

It is of Chinese origin, its popularity spread to various corners of the world, the first was New Zealand, the country where it adopted the name which it is known by today thanks to the native bird whose curious plumage resembles the "hairs" of said fruit as well it is their staple food. Meanwhile, today the cultivation of kiwi is mainly concentrated in countries with a Mediterranean climate like Italy, France, United States, Chile and Argentina.

Belonging to the family of the actinide, kiwi comes from a vine that can reach the height of about 4 meters, whose fruits weigh about 50 to 90 grams, are oval with brown skin covered by fine lint, while the inside is the bright green flesh and tiny black edible seeds arranged around a yellowish heart; sweet taste and a slightly acidic mix reminds one of peach, strawberry and melon's soft and juicy texture. There are more than 400 varieties, of which include: Hayward. It is the best known and most requested green species in the market (present from October to May); can weigh up to 100 grams and has an exquisite taste and excellent quality.

Gold. It is the golden kind, resulting from various crossings made in New Zealand. It is harvested from May to November and skin color dark gold and is not covered with lint. The pulp will have a yellow hue and the taste is sweet with a citrus hint; the aroma smells like a mixture of mango, peach and melon.

Recent Findings

Kiwi is composed mostly of water, so it has few calories (54 calories per 100 grams), but this is not so significant as the results of some research conducted by scientists at the University of Oslo, Norway, which has shown that eating 2 or 3 pieces a day gives the same benefits as taking a tablet of aspirin to improve heart health, as it helps to thin the blood, reducing the formation of clots and reduce blockages causing fat (cholesterol).

In turn, analysis by Rutgers University in the UK, showed that their daily intake can provide important protection against various cancers (esophagus, mouth, stomach, breast, lung and pancreas). Also in this prestigious house of study Dr. Paul Lachance evaluated various fruits to determine which one provides greater nutritional value, finding that among the 27 most consumed kiwi was the top as it contains:

- Vitamin C. One piece covers the daily needs of adults and children, it is beyond the capabilities of orange, also defending the body from infection (colds, flu) and promoting iron absorption which prevents anemia and keeps bones in good condition and blood vessels, as well.

- Potassium. Controls the activity of the heart and works with sodium to maintain fluid balance in the body. Kiwi has (450 milligrams) beating banana (370 milligrams).

- Magnesium. Good for bowel function, nerves, muscles, bones and teeth.

- Vitamin E. Powerful antioxidant that protects cells from the aging process, reduces the risk of heart disease and cancer.

- Folic Acid. Aids in the production of red and white blood cells. Therefore its deficiency can contribute to some problems of anemia, and of particular importance during pregnancy, protecting against birth defects.

- Lutein. Antioxidant that may reduce the risk of macular degeneration related to the elderly. In a recent study they found that these properties in kiwi are above spinach and all other fruits and vegetables, except for yellow corn, in this particular element.

- Fiber. This fruit is an excellent source of dietary fiber, as much soluble (which plays a protective function in heart disease and diabetes) as insoluble, which helps prevent constipation, diverticulitis and hemorrhoids.

Its major component is water. It is moderate in its caloric contribution, because of its amount of carbohydrates.

It's very rich in vitamin C; more than twice that of an orange, and B vitamins, including folic acid. It's also rich in minerals like potassium, magnesium and fiber, soluble and insoluble, with a powerful laxative effect. Fiber improves intestinal transit.

Vitamin C is involved in the formation of collagen, bones and teeth, red blood cells and enhances the absorption of iron from food and resistance to infections. Folic acid works in the production of red and white blood cells in genetic material synthesis and the formation of antibodies in the immune system. Magnesium is related to gut function, nerves and muscles, is part of bones and teeth, improves immunity and has a mild laxative effect. Potassium is required for the generation and transmission of nerve impulses for normal muscle activity and intervenes in water balance in and out of the cell. This goes with skin and all in the smoothie "DRUBINLIFE".

MANGO

Mango, in addition to its pleasant flavor, has endless properties highlighting the contribution of vitamin C, its laxative effect, diuretic and very filling.

Mango is the fruit of a tree (Mangifera indica) that came from Asia to Brazil (XVIII century) thanks to the Portuguese. There are thousands of varieties of mango: green-skinned, reddish or yellowish; round, heart-shaped or bean; a soft pulp or very stringy, etc. It should be eaten on point (neither too ripe nor too green)

Properties of Mango

Its fiber content gives it laxative properties. Fiber prevents or ameliorates constipation, helps to reduce blood cholesterol rate, has good glycemic control and is very satisfying. It has beneficial effects in diabetics and overweight people, of course, in adequate amounts. This is very convenient in cases of cholesterol, obesity and constipation. Therefore, it wouldn't be appropriate for people with diarrhea.

Mango has antioxidant properties thanks to its high level of Vitamin C. It's ideal in cases of degenerative diseases and smokers. Mango is a good alternative for those unable to tolerate other sources of vitamin C such as oranges, peppers, lemons and kiwis. This supply of vitamin C will also collaborate on having a good immune system to defend against infections.

In cases of iron deficiency (anemia) it can collaborate with iron absorption, being that it's rich in vitamin C.

It has a diuretic effect through its potassium contribution. Mango is ideal for people who need to remove fluid (in some cases obesity and hypertension) and do not want to be demineralized. On the other hand, for those who have an excess of potassium (kidney failure, etc.) should avoid it or consult with your doctor.

So from what we've seen, mango also assists in diets to lose weight as it is filling, has a mild laxative effect, rich in nutrients, low in fat, is a diuretic and is used, with the skin, in the smoothie "DRUBINLIFE".

STRAWBERRY:

Strawberry properties, your ally in health

Strawberry is one of the richest fruits and brings you many health benefits both for your body and mood. I'll tell you how to take advantage of their virtues. . .

Strawberry is a fruit that pleases most people. Its sweet flavor and red color distinguish it over any other food. It provides livelihood and vitamin C.

It also contains phyto-nutrients and antioxidants that help combat the dreaded free radicals, which cause many cases of various cancers.

"This is a very versatile fruit. People are not real familiar with its properties and although the price is more expensive than other fruit, it's recommended that you eat strawberries continuously, if you can, as you'll notice the benefits in your body.

You can eat it before meals or as part of a salad accompanied with other vegetables. It is ideal for children over one year old, before one year is not recommended because the baby may have allergies, "There are more than 600 varieties of this fruit which differ in taste, texture, aroma and color. Strawberries that exhibit a deep red color are the sweetest and most chosen by the consumer.

"It's one of the tastiest fruits and provides many benefits to the human body"," Provides protection and prevents both cell structure damage and oxygenation of the cell.

Its properties act as a safeguard for the heart of possible risks and also has an anti-inflammatory effect that is great for the people with muscle problems or bone pain."

Another benefit to consider is that strawberry contains a soluble fiber which facilitates the absorption of carbohydrates and helps maintain blood sugar levels in their balanced state.

Thus, many women who consume it regularly ensure that its intake gives them peace of mind, reduced stress and less pain during their menstrual cycle or during menopause. This was revealed in a survey conducted by the Commission of Strawberries in California.

Its rich flavor, accompanied by the above benefits, are a good choice and should not only be intended for a dessert topping.

Tips for best consumption and conservation of strawberries:

- It should be consumed as soon as it is purchased being that it loses its properties within a matter of days and is a very delicate fruit to keep in the fridge for prolonged time.
- It should not be fed to infants under 1 year as it is highly likely that some sort of intolerance occurs.
- To preserve them they must be removed from the package they come in, placed in a bowl, washed, covered with plastic wrap and stored in the fridge.
- Several people freeze them, but it's not recommended because its properties are easily lost.
- There are various ways of eating them. Ideal for breakfast yogurt, cereal and strawberries or for lunch as part of a salad with other fruits and vegetables
- By consuming only100 grams of this fruit a day will cover the necessary amount of recommended vitamin C.

BANANA:

Bananas or dwarf bananas are an essential part of the daily diet for the inhabitants of over a hundred tropical and subtropical countries.

Its best Season

You can find this delicious and nutritious fruit in the market throughout the year.

How to pick and conserve them

They must always be intact, without bumps or bruises.

In bananas eaten raw, the skin color is indicative of the degree of maturity of the fruit. The ones that are too soft must be discarded.

The presence of spots and dots, black or brown, on the skin does not affect the quality of the fruit.

This fruit does not require special storage conditions, just keep them in a cool, dry place protected from direct sun light. If kept in the refrigerator, the will blacken so that its external appearance is impaired, but this in no way affects its nutritional quality. The darkening of the skin can be avoided if wrapped in newspaper

Dwarf bananas are better preserved when they stay in their bunch and not when they are by themselves and are to be consumed as soon as possible once they have reached their maturity. They shouldn't be refrigerated...

Nutritional Properties

It is distinguished by its carbohydrate content, therefore its caloric value is high. The most known nutrients of the banana are potassium, magnesium, folic acid and astringent action substances; not neglecting the high amount of fiber, however.

The latter makes it an appropriate fruit for those suffer from diarrheal diseases. Potassium is a necessary mineral for the generation and transmission of nerve impulses and normal muscle activity, it's also involved in water balance inside and out of the cell. Magnesium is related to bowel operation, nerves and muscles, forms part of bones and teeth, enhances immunity and has a mild laxative effect. Folic acid is intervenes in the production of red and white blood cells, in genetic material synthesis and in the formation of antibodies in the immune system. As well, it helps to treat or prevent anemia and spine bifida in pregnancy.

Mix all of this with apple juice, all means everything even the skin (except for avocado, mango, banana and the apple seeds. . .) And take it every morning before breakfast after the first two glasses of water that you should drink when you rise . . . now that you know the properties of these ingredients go and prepare a Drubinlife and continue reading your book. During the morning between 7:00 a.m. and 9:00 a.m. is the best time for absorption of nutrients in the small intestine, it is the perfect time to have breakfast. If you're sick breakfast should be earlier, before 6:30 am. Breakfast before 7:30 am is very beneficial for those who want to stay fit.

Those who always skip breakfast should change their habit, it is less harmful to eat breakfast between 9:00 am and 10:00 am rather than not do it at all.

Drubinlife is a full breakfast, we'll explain later how to complete the meals of the day.

(Here I will share several emails which came to me during the preparation of my book that can be very useful as well.)

Going to Bed and Waking Up Early

9pm - 11pm: is the time in which the body performs removal activities where unnecessary and toxic chemicals are detoxified through the lymphatic system of the body. This time of day should be used to find a state of relaxation, listening to music, for example.

Usually by this time people perform activities such as cleaning the kitchen, make sure everything is ready for the activities of the next day, etc. activities that generate the state of a lack of relaxation which in turn generates a negative health effect.

11pm - 1:00 a.m.: the body performs the detoxification of the liver and ideally this should be done in a state of deep sleep.

During the early morning hours of 1:00 a.m. to 3:00 a.m. is the detox process of the gallbladder. Ideally, this should also happen in a state of deep sleep.

Early morning 3:00 a.m. to 5:00 a.m. is the detoxification of the lungs. That is why sometimes during these hours it can produce excess of severe cough. When the detoxification process has reached the respiratory tract it's best not to take cough medicine as it interferes with the process of removing toxins.

In the morning between 5:00 a.m. to 7:00 a.m. is the colon detox, it is the time of going to bathroom to empty the bowel.

During the morning between 7:00 a.m. to 9:00 a.m. is when the absorption of nutrients in the small intestine is prime, therefore, the perfect time to have breakfast. If you're sick breakfast should be eaten earlier, before 6:30 a.m. Breakfast before 7:30 am is very beneficial for those who want to stay in shape. Those who always skip breakfast should try to change that habit, at least by eating breakfast between 9 a.m. and 10 a.m. instead of not eating at all.

Going to bed late and waking up late will disrupt the removal process of unnecessary chemicals in your body. In addition to that, you should keep in mind that between 12 a.m. & 4 a.m. is the time in which the bone marrow produces blood in your bones, therefore, try to sleep well and do not go to sleep late.

TAKE CARE OF YOUR HEALTH

Live life without limits!

Share this information with people you care about. Recommend them this book to gain health and energy every day.

The "top five" cancer causing foods

1. **Hotdogs**
   Because they are high in nitrates, "Cancer Prevention Coalition" warns that children should not eat more than 12 hot dogs in a month. If you cannot live without them, buy hotdogs which are made WITHOUT sodium nitrate, but it's better to not eat them.

2. **Processed meats and bacon**
   These also contain high levels of sodium nitrate like hotdogs, other content in bacon and other processed meats also increase the risk of heart disease. Saturated fat in bacon is also a great contributor to the generation of cancer.

3. **Donuts**
   Doughnuts are double cancer-causing. First, because drowned in fluoride, refined sugar and hydrogenated oil and then fried at high temperatures. Donuts are the #1 "Food" of all which most increases the risk of cancer.

4. **Fried Potatoes**
   Like donuts, French fries are made with hydrogenated oils and then cooked at high temperatures. Also, they contain

acrylamides that are generated during the process of high temperature cooking. They should be called cancer fries instead of French fries.

5. **Snacks and cookies or famous snacks-chips**
   These are usually made with fluoride and sugar. Even their labels are proudly presented as free of trans fats usually they contain them just in lesser amounts.

The 5 causes of death from cancer in USA

1. Lung Cancer
2. Colon Cancer
3. Pancreas
4. Prostate
5. Mammary gland

BRAIN DAMAGING HABITS (kill neurons)

1. **Not eating breakfast**
   People who skip breakfast have low blood sugar. This leads to an insufficient supply of nutrients to the brain causing its gradual degeneration.

2. **Overeating**
   This causes hardening of the brain arteries, causing, besides this, low mental capacity.

3. **Smoking**
   It causes brain diminution and further promotes Alzheimer and others like: cancer, aging, toxins, etc.

4. **Consuming high amounts of sugar**
   The high consumption of sugar will interrupt the absorption of proteins and nutrients resulting in malnutrition and may interfere with brain development.

5. **Air Pollution**
   The brain is the largest oxygen consumer in our body. Inhaling polluted air decreases the supply of oxygen decreasing cerebral efficiency.

6. **Little sleep**
   Sleep allows our brain to rest. Lack of sleep for extended periods of time accelerates loss of brain cells.

7. **Sleeping with our head covered**
   Sleeping with our head covered increases the concentration of carbon dioxide and oxygen is decreased causing adverse effects to our brain.

8. **Working your brain during illness**
   Besides the difficulty for the brain to respond while sick, working and studying also damage it.

9. **Lack of stimulation**
   Thinking is the best way to stimulate our brain not doing so causes the brain to shrink and therefore, its capacity too.

10. **Practice Intelligent Conversation**
    Deep or intellectual conversations promote cerebral efficiency. The same goes for reading good books.

Leading causes that damage the liver

1. Going to sleep late and waking up late
2. Not urinating in the morning
3. Overeating
4. Skipping breakfast
5. Consuming a lot of medication
6. Consuming preservatives, colorings, artificial sweeteners
7. Consuming unhealthy cooking oils. Reduce, as much as you can, the consumption of fried foods even if you use healthy

oils. Do not consume fried foods when you are tired or sick unless you are real skinny, but if you can avoid it.
8. Consuming raw or overcooked foods will add additional load on the liver.

Vegetables should be eaten raw or a little cooked. If you consume fried vegetables you should do it in one sitting, that is to say don't save them for later consumption (left overs). We just have to adopt a healthier lifestyle and better eating habits. Keeping good eating habits and exercise is great for our body to absorb what it needs and eliminate chemicals on its own "schedule".

TAKE YOUR HEALTH SERIOUS. . . . and share this information with everyone who you love, share with them Drubinlife.

Margarine and Butter: interesting and incredible

Margarine was originally manufactured to fatten turkeys when what they actually did was kill them.

People who had put up the money for research wanted to recover it, so they started to think of a way to do it.

It was a white substance that had no appeal as being edible, so they added the yellow coloring and sold it to people instead of butter.

How about that? . . .

Now they have released some new flavors to sell more of it to suckers like you and me.

Do you know the difference between margarine and butter?

Keep reading until the end…because it gets pretty interesting!

Comparison between butter and margarine:

Both have the same amount of calories.

Butter is slightly higher in saturated fats at 8 grams compared to 5 grams in margarine.

Eating margarine instead of butter can increase your risk of coronary heart disease by 53% in women, according to a recent medical study at the University of Harvard.

Eating butter increases the absorption of many nutrients found in other foods.

Butter has many nutritional benefits where margarine only has a few which are added in the process of making it. Butter tastes much better than margarine and it can enhance the taste of other foods.

Butter has been around for centuries where margarine has been around less than 100 years. Now, about margarine: It is very high in trans fatty acids. (Yes, these fatty acids have just recently been found, by scientists, to be triple the risk coronary diseases. It increases total cholesterol and LDL (bad cholesterol) and lowers HDL (good cholesterol).

It increases fivefold the risk of cancer.

It lowers the quality of breast milk, decreases the immunological reaction in the body and decreases insulin reaction.

And here's the most disturbing factor:

Margarine is ONE MOLECULE shy of being PLASTIC!

This fact alone is sufficient to avoid the use of margarine for life and anything else that is hydrogenated (this means that hydrogen is added, which changes the molecular structure of substances).

You can try this yourself: purchase a little margarine and leave it in your garage or a shaded area. Within a few days you will notice two things: there will be no flies; not even those little pesky bugs will go near it (that should tell you something). It does not rot or start to smell bad because it has no nutritional value.

Nothing grows in it. Even those teeny weeny microorganisms can't grow in it. Why? Because it is nearly plastic!!

Would you melt Tupperware and spread it on a Toast?

We can also add that if we take a piece of margarine and put it on the grill or on a griddle for cooking steaks, it produces black smoke!

After alcohol abuse comes the hangover.

After drinking too much during a festive day, it's common to suffer the inevitable hangover the next day. He who has had too much alcohol is cannot avoid the classic symptoms: the head seems like it's going to explode, dizziness, inability to concentrate, physical weakness and extreme thirst. In short, the body is battered, basically because the body reverses the glucose to metabolize alcohol; Glucose is sugar and sugar is energy. The result is that we are weakened in all aspects.

Too much alcohol also attacks the central nervous system, and provokes drowsiness and irritation; it corrupts the chemical mechanisms of the brain and causes headaches. It irritates the mucous membrane of the digestive apparatus, causes nausea, vomiting and even diarrhea. It inhibits the action of the antidiuretic hormone, causing thirst and dry mouth. But that's not all.

Excessive alcohol intake enhances weight gain and accumulation of fat in the abdomen. "The permanent consumption can cause brain damage, Type 2 diabetes, ulcers and inflammation in the stomach and intestine, hepatitis, depression, lesions to the kidneys, bladder, prostate and pancreas, among other ailments."

How to avoid a hangover? Useful tips for those who drink liquor and have not been able to leave it, even though my best counsel is not to consume alcohol at all. These tips are for those who will continue drinking alcohol even though you know how harmful it is.

1. Although a hangover is unavoidable, if you drink a lot of alcohol, it can be even worse if distilled in a mixture of fruit juice drinks, as with whiskey generates more discomfort when mixed with other substances.
2. Alcohol and cigarettes are a nefarious duo for the body: the more nicotine the less amount of oxygen in the blood and the intoxication of the body is generated faster.

How to relieve hangover, a little.

1. The main cause of a hangover is dehydration caused by alcohol, a potent diuretic that stimulates the loss of fluid in the body. Fill yourself with water before, during and after your night of drinking. Before bedtime drink water as to help your body metabolize alcohol and rid itself of toxins. Citrus juices such as lemon and orange are excellent because they have antioxidants, protectors and vitamin C which enter the body. Drink isotonics to replenish mineral salts and don't forget coconut water, rich in potassium.
2. Avoid black coffee to ward off the hangover, as it is a drink which also has diuretic properties, namely that further dehydrated body.
3. Eat easily digestible foods to lighten the load of the organism since it's forced to process excess alcohol. "To reduce the effects of hangovers opt for light food, low in fat, rich in fruits, vegetables and liquids (such as drubinlife or V10) ". Include in the menu light crackers and savory breads. Alcohol

increases the acidity and irritates stomach mucus; salted and dried food slows acid production, and also strengthens the liver for processing toxins from alcohol. On the other hand, avoid yellow cheese and fried

4. Although there are some medications on the market that promise to minimize physical damage caused by alcohol (combined antacid, analgesic and antiemetic, which prevents feeling sick), none of them are able to solve all the consequences of drunkenness.

5. Wherever it passes, alcohol causes problems. In the brain it acts on neurons, causing disinhibition first and then lethargy. Five hours after alcohol intake brain cells begin to recover, but remain highly sensitive; making light and noise bothersome. The following day damages are not yet repaired and that's why it is so difficult regain focus. Rest: keep the light out, the curtains closed and stay in bed. At times like this the body asks for rest.

6. Some herbs help the liver cells to renew and accelerate the detoxification process. Herbal teas (no caffeine) facilitate the process. Juices mixed with orange and lemon help replenish the body's strength and the mixture of passion fruit, coconut water and ginger, in a blender, results in a tasty product and at the same time helps to liberate yourself from the hangover symptoms. Another ideal combination is that of orange, banana, pineapple and carrot, Drubinlife, V10. Any juices mentioned here will be a perfect complement after a night of drinks. (my advice will always be don't drink if you love yourself)

Theories of Aging: Free Radicals

Keep in mind that aging is considered a multifactorial process that represents a gradual deterioration of physiological functions of homeostasis and allostasis. Of the many developed and investigated theories, one of the most currently accepted fulfills the requirements that are required to explain the aging process

(Universal: the associated process that must occur to varying degrees in all individuals of a species. *Intrinsic:* endogenous causes, which do not depend on extrinsic factors. *Progressive:* occur during the development of life. *Deterioration:* considered only as part of the aging process, is the free radical theory of aging.

It is proposed that the free radicals formed by metabolizing residual toxicity from oxygen derivatives (and other oxidizing agents such as reactive nitrogen species) are responsible for any damages associated with the cells and thereby cause aging, generating highly reactive molecular fragments which can lead to very disruptive reactions and degenerative processes such as cancer, atherosclerosis, amyloidosis and immunodeficiency, decrease antioxidant levels and deterioration of repaired damages. It is oxidative damage to the cell, in reality, it is oxygen poisoning which dooms all aerobic organisms.

Origin of the free radical theory as the cause of aging

The first time the theory of free radicals was postulated was in 1950 by Harman, who returns to retouch the theory later in 1972. There are many experiments and groups of scientists with different evidence which supports this theory as one of the causing factors of aging. In order to defend this theory we must demonstrate that since we have good anti-oxidation systems, even beneficial for determined metabolic routes by intermediate molecules which are generated (it's like two sides of the same coin, one side is beneficial and other destructive).

Under conditions of in vitro, different studies demonstrate how the oxidizing effects can be counteracted by the application of antioxidants. Under live conditions, these antioxidant systems are unable to counteract all free radicals continuously generated during the life of the cell. At specific times the accumulated free radicals increase, purely physiological moments, which are resolved in a timely manner. It is the single accumulation throughout the cell life which is a matter of concern and study on theories of aging.

Free radical damage at the cellular level

Free radicals pose cell damage and result in tissue damage, affecting the performance of the organs. Damage will occur at the DNA level, with consequent worsening in terms of protein production and injuries to membrane lipids, altering the fluidity and thereby hindering good communication within and between cells. We'll have, therefore, damage both structurally and functionally of the cell (molecule signals for growth, apoptosis and neurotransmission). It implies a worsening of the organism to respond to stress and maintain homeostasis (response to oxidative stress, heat shock, radiation, alkylating agents, heavy metals, etc.)

It has been seen that in old animals there is greater oxidation accumulation than in young animals, counting protein, oxidized lipids and DNA. Increased life span also causes to increase the rate of free radicals involved in degenerative diseases.

Free radicals and mitochondrial theory

In the theory of aging because of free radicals, one must include the mitochondrial aging theory, since it is this organelle within the cell, the main producer of ROS (reactive oxygen species) and (NO) Nitric oxide is also responsible for oxidation. There are other cellular organelles (peroxisomes, microsomes) also generators of ROS in which must be added in the presence of certain transition metal complexes which may react with each other giving place for more radicals.

Mitochondria is the principal source of endogenous oxidizing involved in aging. Reactive oxygen species are continuously generated in the electron transport chain in mitochondria. The production is cumulative, which gradually results in chronic oxidative stress. The more the respiration rate the more the possibilities of accumulating reactive oxygen species (ROS).

It has been found that those cells in the process of mitotic forming have not yet been fully defined in its functionality (cells protected against aging by moderate oxygen consumption and regeneration of mitochondria that accompanies the mitosis), occur less in reactive species than in those where the cell is mature and differentiated. Here the transportation chain of electrons and cellular respiration by mitochondria have to operate at full capacity to synthesize sufficient ATP required for the specific function of the cell. We find high specificity in muscle including the heart, liver and nervous system cells. Oxidation production by mitochondria is the key that determines the maximum potential longevity.

The mitochondrial theory has been tested by several laboratories. Note that mitochondria are not only involved in the aging structure level but also in functionality level. It has been observed that mitochondrial activity decreases with age affecting, as noted earlier, especially liver, muscle and brain.

Many laboratories are more interested in studying the biomarkers of oxidative stress than to study the amount of oxidant production. Some biomarkers study two: ethane and pentane for lipid peroxidation, protein oxidation and the DNA oxidation. Mitochondrial DNA is more affected by ROS than nuclear, since it is in continuous exposure to it and they do not have histone and protection mechanisms as do the nuclear. This increases the rate of mtDNA mutations, leading to the deterioration of the function of aerobic respiration mtDNA encodes proteins as a respiratory chain). Less electron transfer production leads to increased ROS production, thus establishing a vicious cycle between oxidative stress and decreased energy.

All this can block mitochondrial division and renewal organelle, and lead to a self-destruction process (digestion autophagy of mitochondria, thus decreasing ATP production and proteins necessary for specialized cell work and aging pigment accumulation: lipofuscin, also aggravated by the accumulation of dysfunctional lysosomes which leads to irremediable cell death.

Chlorophyll

It is well known that chlorophyll molecules are necessary for the process of photosynthesis by which light is transformed into energy, but has recently its antioxidant properties have been discovered. Chlorophyll produced by plants is soluble; while that which is chemically altered and is the basis of products sold in pharmacies is water soluble. This means the second is more difficult to be absorbed by the gastrointestinal system. Moreover, the soluble chlorophyll amplifies its antioxidant property because it contains beta carotene.

These antioxidants are found in all green plants and fresh fruits.

If you've tried diets and exercise programs without achieving desired results, today I'll give you the solution so that you can finally lose weight without having to diet but exercise, yes!

Diets and exercise fail because they make you lose water weight that your body has accumulated! None of these diets or exercises actually focus on burning fat that is within your body. For that reason, when you stop the diet, your weight goes right back up. Also, your body creates more fat trying to fight off toxins that your body accumulates that's why if you don't detoxify your body you cannot lose the fat from your body.

To burn fat, you need to use a colon cleanser to purify your body and turn it into a fat burning furnace!

Over the years, your body has accumulated food, fats, plaque and other things in the digestive system. When these things accumulate they cause your body to function in a different way. Your body works harder to digest and process the food you eat; the fat, plaque and other things stick to your intestines and colon and you get fat.

Sure, you might wonder how it is that this makes you gain weight. Well, it's simple. When these things are stuck in your bowel and colon, your body gets fewer vitamins and nutrients from the food you eat. So that your body gets the right amount of vitamins and nutrients the brain sends a signal to your stomach that it is hungry. Your brain tells your stomach to feel hungry, this is so that you eat more food and you obtain more vitamins and nutrients.

So, you eat more food or eat more times a day. Now, the negative thing in this is that when you eat you not only receive food and nutrients the body needs but you also get the calories from the food!!! So you gain weight because you consume more calories than your body needs. The calories that your body can not burn quickly turn into fat that accumulates around the body with the majority sticking in the abdomen area. But don't lose hope.

Did you know that the reason most people fail with diets is because they cannot follow it for an extended time? The reason for this is that diets rob your body of the energy it needs from vitamins and nutrients. If you lack these, you're going to feel anxiety, despair and suffer from nervousness. This is because your body lacks the vitamins and nutrients you were consuming before!

With drubinlife it's like being on a diet, but you will not fail because drubinlife contains all the vitamins and nutrients your body needs to function without problems. The high antioxidant concentration will boost your metabolism and make it work better. The metabolism is responsible for burning fat throughout the day and when you sleep. The metabolism is more active at the time you're taking drubinlife, your metabolism will be active for more time and not just for when you eat. To view the results yourself start preparing your drubinlife every morning now.

How a natural colon cleanse works?

A colon cleanse is going to remove all the putrefaction that gets stuck in the walls of your colon and intestines. It is estimated that one has 5-15 kilos of fat, plaque and other things that are stuck in your digestive system. The colon cleanse will not cause you to have diarrhea like a laxative does.

When all the putrefaction is loose, your digestive system will be able to consume meals more easily. Your body will be able to extract completely vitamins and nutrients of meals. You will eat less because your brain will recognize that it has all vitamins and nutrients the body needs.

When you get rid of all this from your body, you will notice a difference in weight of 5-15 kilos because all you had stuck will have left your body. This is what is stuck in your digestive system. Do not expect that it just leaves your body all at once. It will come out gradually in a healthy manner. If it is removed all at the same time your body can have a negative reaction such as excessive tiredness. But with the colon cleanse, it will be removed gently and healthily and you will you'll feel better, have more energy and be healthier!

There are many ways to detoxify naturally. In one day (24hrs) eating broccoli and drinking only water. Although, there many companies offering a variety of products for this process and they do work, but I just limit myself to natural ways that you can do in home naturally and safely, of course consult, before making any nutritional changes, with your doctor to give you approval.

There are naturopathic treatments such as rectal enemas where with a bag of warm water with piece of wormwood, a teaspoon of activated carbon, half of a lemon and a cup of black coffee in a bulb syringe or an enema bag. It's a great liver drainer, but should only be applied through the rectum, not ingesting it orally. Rectally, so as to clean with just 1 to 2 liters of water and to clean the intestine wall, getting rid of the putrefaction which doesn't allow the absorption of food.

Conclusion

The colon cleanse will clean everything from your intestine and colon. This will cause your body to consume all the vitamins and nutrients with ease! This will make you lose weight because you will not carry the weight that you had stuck. The products should be natural so that you don't have side effects with other medicines that you may be taking.

Energy Drinks

Energy Drinks is dangerous as it contains caffeine, ginseng and guarana (all legal stimulants), sugars, artificial sweeteners, taurine (an amino acid said to lower blood pressure). **Energy Drinks** promises increased energy, better concentration, yield sharper cognition, better strength, higher metabolism, faster reaction time. **Energy Drinks** offers: increased heart rate, increased blood pressure, anxiety, apprehension, hyperactivity, insomnia, hypoglycemia, dehydration. One can of **Energy Drinks** or any other "energy drink" increases the risk of heart attack or stroke. Soda pop laden with caffeine causes blood to be stickier and become a pre-cursor to cardiovascular problems. One hour after drinking a **Energy Drinks**, the blood system becomes abnormal, functioning as it would in a patient with heart disease. This effect is even seen in younger people. Take a look at the Red Bull website. The company has aligned itself - through high-dollar sponsorships, which are nothing more than manipulative campaign advertising - with the sports crowd. It began with rodeo; the **Energy Drinks** logo is tailor-made for a cowboy character. You will find a superstar athlete wearing the **Energy Drinks** logo in stadiums and venues worldwide. But to suggest that athletes will benefit from the "energy" **Energy Drinks** offers is wildly irresponsible and wrong.

Unlike rehydration electrolyte balance in Gatorade, **Energy Drinks** is filled shock stimulants causing rapid dehydration, energy drinks are doing exceptional danger when used in rigorous physical activities. Loss of consciousness, kidney failure and death are some of the results of greater concern of severe dehydration. Even mild dehydration makes you feel foggy and slow - not improving physical or mental performance for anyone. Combining the health threat of **Energy Drinks** powerful stimulants with a heavy depressant can lead to heart failure and other health crises. Norway, France, Denmark and Uruguay have even banned sales of **Energy Drinks** completely. History has taught us that we cannot expect responsible behavior from companies. They have an apparent duty to shareholders to make money without obstacles for ethical considerations. That's why the Food and Drug Administration has been named our faithful watchman.

"**Energy Drinks** was created to stimulate the brain in people subjected to great physical exertion and in a "stress coma" and never to be consumed like an innocent, refreshing drink.

It was created by Dietrich Mateschitz, an industrialist of Austrian origin who discovered the drink by chance.

It happened during a business trip to Hong Kong, while working for a toothbrush manufacturer. The liquid, based on a formula that contained caffeine and taurine, caused rage in that country.

Precisely, he imagined a huge success of this drink in Europe, where the product did not exist, besides he saw it was a chance to become an entrepreneur.

BUT THE TRUTH ABOUT THIS DRINK IS ANOTHER THING: FRANCE and DENMARK have just prohibited it as a cocktail of death due to its mixed components of vitamins "GLUCURONOLACTONE" a highly hazardous chemical, which was developed by the Department of Defense of the United

States during the 60's to boost the morale of the troops based in VIETNAM, which acted like a hallucinogenic drug that calmed the stress of war. But its effects on the organism were so devastating, that it was discontinued because of the many cases of migraines, cerebral tumors and liver disease, which shown in the soldiers who consumed it.

And despite this, on the can of **Energy Drinks** it still reads, among their components: GLUCURONOLACTONE, cataloged medically as a stimulant.

But what it doesn't say on the can of **Energy Drinks** are the consequences of consumption, which we're obligated to place a series of WARNINGS:

1. It is dangerous to take it if you do not exercise, and its energizing function accelerates the heart rate and can cause a massive heart attack.

You run the risk of suffering a cerebral hemorrhage, because **Energy Drinks** contains components that dilute the blood so that it takes much less work for the heart to pump blood, and so it's able to deliver physical force with less effort.

It is prohibited to mix **Energy Drinks** with alcohol, because the mixture turns the drink into a "Deadly Bomb" that directly attacks the liver, causing the affected area to never regenerate again.

One of the main components of **Energy Drinks** is vitamin B12, used in medicine to help patients which are in a coma recover; hence the pressure and excited state in which you find yourself after taking it is like being in a drunk state.

The regular consumption of **Energy Drinks** triggers an occurrence of a number of neurological diseases and irreversible neuronal

CONCLUSION:

It is a drink that should be prohibited in Mexico, Venezuela, Dominican Republic, Puerto Rico and other countries in the Caribbean as other nations are already starting to mix it with alcohol and making a time bomb for the human body, primarily among adolescents and adults ignorant because of their lack of experience.

REPORT by Ph. D. Khalet Gebara, MD, UCLA University, California, USA:

11 hour days are bad for the heart.

People who work 10 or 11 hours a day are more likely to suffer serious heart problems, including heart attacks, than those who work 7 to 8 hours.

The highest incidence of heart problems among those working overtime was independent of a range of other risk factors including smoking, being overweight or being high in cholesterol.

More fundamental, long hours may be associated with job-related stress, which interferes with metabolic processes. Indeed these are the evils of this new century.

HOW TO ELIMINATE TOXINS FROM THE BODY: (PART III)- How does waste produces disease?

To understand how the presence of waste in the body can make you sick, remember that the body is a bunch of cells, which work because all these cells are active.

Cells, as a group, form our bodies, which by themselves lack organs which allow them to breathe, produce energy, eliminate wastes, reproduce and send or receive messages. Cells are the smallest "units of life" that we have, but, nevertheless, they are completely dependent on the environment in which they find themselves. By not being able to travel, oxygen and nutrients they need to be supplied to them and the waste they produce, removed. Body fluids such as blood, lymph and cell serum, are responsible for this transportation. Formerly, these organic liquids were called humors and spoke of the humoral fluids state. Now they have changed the words and is spoken of "organic space."

70% of our body is made of liquid. Our cells are literally submerged in an interior ocean comprised of cellular fluid whose current circulates nurturing and purifying the blood and lymph streams. This liquid composition, therefore, is essential for cells because it represents their living environment.

If you were to extend cell tissues, it would cover an area of 200 hectares. A hundred kilometers of blood vessels serve as channels to irrigate this huge area. However, our body has only a few liters of blood. How can our cells survive with such a restricted nutrient liquid? Two factors compensate for the lack of fluid. First, the capillaries are not all filled at the same time, only the most active parts of the body get an abundant irrigation: the digestive organs when eat, the brain when we think, the muscles when we perform work which requires force. Moreover, the speed of circulation compensates for the lack of liquid, when circulating at a high speed in a closed system as the circulatory system, the blood often and quickly returns to the same sites. It takes approximately one minute or so for the blood to make a full round in the body.

Differentiated irrigation and circulation velocity allows for the correct irrigation of every cell. But there is a third and essential factor that adds to the other two: the cells can function normal because these organic liquids are clean. In effect, if such small quantities of liquids can be used to ensure nutrition and debugging such a large amount of cells, it's because these liquids consistently retain their ideal composition, i.e. they are not overloaded with waste.

Therefore, one of the main tasks of the body is maintaining the purity of the organic liquids. However, the fifty billion cells that make up the body excrete humoral waste into the environment as if it were a sewer, and five to seven million dead cells are dumped each day in to the blood and lymph. Moreover, as we have seen, multiple poisons penetrate our body through the respiratory, digestive tract and skin.

To maintain the purity of its inner environment, the body has several emunctories (organ or duct that removes waste from the body). Each in its own way, liver, intestines, kidneys, sweat and sebaceous glands, just as with respiratory system filters waste and removes it outward. When these organs are working normally and production and waste input is not high, the process remains clean and cells can function properly.

Conversely when wastes are abundant and emunctories are lazy or deficient, the system gradually accumulates waste and the organic situation is degraded. The blood thickens, it becomes more dense and heavy, and no longer circulates as easily through the blood vessels. Waste transported through the blood penetrates the lymph and the cell fluid. The longer it is clogged with debris the dirtier the liquids will be. Over time, the cells may be embedded in a true swamp, which will paralyze any exchange. The contributions of oxygen and nutrients cannot reach the cells and causes serious deprivation. When the waste isn't transported and is rejected by the cells the degree of surrounding pollution will increase even more. In these conditions, cells can no longer perform their job and neither can the bodies composed of them. Its activity decreases and then it is interrupted, to a greater or lesser degree.

When waste is deposited on blood vessel walls, it reduces the diameter thereof, which further retards the circulation speed, irrigation of tissues and the interchanges. When it accumulates, litter and debris clog the emunctory filter, congesting organs and blocking joints. When tissues become irritated, inflamed and hardened then come a host of different diseases, depending on which organs have been affected and to what degree.

SOURCE: How to Eliminate Toxins from the Body

Processed meat increases the risk of ovarian cancer. Women who eat large amounts of processed meat, such as salami and hot dogs, are at high risk of developing ovarian cancer.

On the other hand, those who consume fish have a low risk of developing the disease.

"This suggests that if dietary guidelines are met to reduce the consumption of processed meats and increase the consumption of poultry and fish, women will reduce the risk of developing ovary cancer."

Most studies by the American Cancer Society on the risk of ovarian cancer focused on the exposure to estrogen throughout the life of a woman.

This means those who begin puberty early and delay getting to menopause have a higher risk of developing the disease.

"Few dietary risk factors were identified for this highly fatal cancer."

It is unknown why processed meats and fish would have an effect on the risk of developing ovarian cancer.

"Processed meat contains substances that might harm the cells and, therefore, cause cancer.

In contrast, omega 3 fatty acids, found in fish fat, are good for your health and are anti-carcinogen," processed meats preserved with nitrites and nitrates can cause nitrosamines, substances that cause cancer in animals.

"But we know that there are other benefits associated with the consumption of white meat and fish, so I think that women should try to have a healthy diet that includes less processed meat and more poultry and fish"

"This would have several benefits and would reduce the risk of developing ovarian cancer," he added.

The results are consistent with the dietary recommendations of the American Cancer Society: reduce consumption of processed meats and red meats, and eat fruits and assorted vegetables.

He assured that there are good reasons to reduce the consumption of red and processed meats, such as reducing the risk of developing heart disease and colon cancer.

"It would be wise to leave processed meats alone except on occasional get togethers, instead of consuming them habitually" SOURCE: American Journal of Clinical Nutrition, printed and online April 14th 2010

Stress triggers symptoms of intestinal disease

People with Inflammatory Bowel Disease (IBD) think that stress can cause the symptoms and a new study makes their inclination correct.

Researchers in Canada found that among 552 patients with intestinal disease, studied for one year, found that the risk of suffering a recurrence of symptoms grew especially when they were stressed.

IBD is a group of disorders characterized by chronic bowel inflammation and symptoms such as abdominal pain and diarrhea. The major disorders are Crohn's disease and ulcerative colitis.

The exact cause of these diseases is unknown, but there would exist an excessive immune system response that damages its own intestinal tissue. Stress does not cause IBD, but is one of the environmental factors that could trigger symptoms in some people.

Previous studies have shown that many people with IBD feel that stress worsens their symptoms, but there is little scientific evidence to support it.

"This is one of the first evidences that the perception of stress has a direct relationship to the disease"

There are biological reasons to believe that response to stress can trigger or aggravate symptoms of IBD.

The sympathetic nervous system that is activated by stress acts on the lining of the colon and exacerbates inflammation. There is evidence that stress hormones could help harmful bacteria settle in the intestines which may aggravate the symptoms.

If stress triggers the symptoms of IBD, it's possible that by learning to manage it better helps prevent it.

The Milk Dilemma

Milk consumption is as old as the first human communities. People have drunk it for centuries as an important part of the daily diet. However, at the present time the question of whether milk is beneficial or not is the subject of scientific research and even advertising campaigns of some organizations.

One fact is undeniable: Milk is a very complete food, especially for children and adolescents. It has a lot of calcium, proteins and vitamins B2, B6 and B12, essential in the metabolic processes and growth. Recent studies show positive connections between health and milk consumption, "Bioactive peptides that are present in it could contribute to a healthy intestinal flora and lower blood pressure."

Other investigators, however, warn of the negative influence that milk consumption may have on health. American Doctor. Alan Goldhammer, founder of TrueNorth Health Education Center, says in his article "Nobody needs milk"

To consume milk and dairy products is a "devastating practice." No other component of the diet causes more pain and suffering-including premature death and disabilities-such as dairy products. Milk can influence in the development of diseases such as diabetes, constipation, otitis, rhinitis, dermatitis, asthma, digestive irritation, arthritis, leukemia and obesity, among others.

However, a study by doctors at the Durand Hospital, in Buenos Aires, Argentina, concluded that milk consumption in children reduces the risk of developing type 2 diabetes and from suffering heart disease in adulthood. The research, which included a group of 365 children and adolescents between 5 and 14 years old, showed that those who consumed milk often had less insulin resistance, ate more fruits and vegetables, and were more active than those who did not include it in their daily diet.

With these pros and cons we are in the same boat as when we began: Is it beneficial or not to drink milk? Apparently, the answer differs according to the physiological characteristics of each person. If you are intolerant to lactose, for example, milk will bring you more disorders than benefits.

Also, the advice from naturopathic doctors is to replace it for soy milk or almond milk or coconut water; all of these have organic proteins which are healthier, without the effect of the lactose.

The right amount is, again, the key. Dairy remains a key link in the food pyramid, but although milk has important nutrients, you don't want to consume a gallon day, because it also contains saturated fats that can raise the cholesterol in the body.

Training without gym equipment (at home): Love your abs! flatten your belly, slim your thighs, and become firm; Exercise at home where you just need music, a wall, a chair, a bucket with water and maybe yoga mat at home allowing you to stay fit and healthy which will raise your self-esteem, also, you'll need to walk or jog if your body allows for it and if the weather is rainy and you can't leave the house, walking or jogging in place or doing some Zumba will work. Unless you can afford a gym pass. Today with the internet you can do to do many exercises for the entire body.

Do not skip breakfast being that fiber in the morning means less hunger in the late afternoon, when it is more likely you feel tired. My morning dose consists of cut oats, usually mixed with flaxseed, raisins and nuts. An early start on eating also keeps your metabolism more active throughout the day; breakfast eaters are thinner than people who just rush out the door. Seven hours of sleep a night not only helps you live longer, but also reduces stress, betters memory and reduces anxiety to eat late at night. Set a bedtime and stick to it.

My goal is 10: 30 pm. Record the final programs and then watch them the next day while pedaling a stationary bike. Admire your work. Turn around and take a look at your stool, which speaks volumes about your intestines and overall health. Your stool should be smooth and S-shaped, like your colon. If it comes out too lumpy, or drops into the bowl like marbles, you're constipated. Increase the intake of fiber and water. This is what happens to me when I travel, so the fiber loading before a trip avoids irritation of the colon. But you do not need Metamucil – here I teach 17 great tasting ways to add fiber to your diet (drubinlife). Don't pamper a back bad, also don't abuse it, staying in your bed only makes it worse. Recent research shows that bed rest weakens the back muscles and prolongs suffering.

Married men can suffer more than active single men only because of all the hedonism. But the best solution is to get up, take a pain reliever and be a soldier. The taste of foods with rich colors are bright more pleasant. They are also full of flavonoids and carotenoids, potent compounds that attach to harmful free radicals in your body, reducing inflammation. Eat 4 colorful fruits, 6 vegetables and fruits each day and you will enjoy the benefits without having to give up other foods. It reminds me that these foods are often more potent than the drugs sold in pharmacies and drugstores.

"Peanut butter is a little higher in fat" Only that it's the type that is good for you which is the mono-unsaturated fat. "Researchers have predicted that the peanut diet could reduce the risk of heart-disease. Just don't go nutty plastering the tasty spread, since it is high in calories.

MORE: 11 ways to load up on lean protein

2. Watermelon. Up to the age of 55, more men suffer from high blood pressure than women. Research suggests that foods rich in potassium can reduce the risk of high blood pressure. Evidence is convincing the authorities so much that the drug administration is allowing food labels to carry a health claim about the connection between food rich in potassium and blood pressure. "There is no dietary requirement for potassium," only a good goal is to take about 2000 milligrams or more a day. "Watermelon, one rich source of this mineral, has more potassium - magnesium 664mg - in one large slice than the amount found in a banana or a cup of orange juice. Cut another slice and enjoy the taste of summer.

Food for Women

1. **Papaya**. This tropical fruit has twice the vitamin C of an orange. Add it to your arsenal against bile, gallbladder disease, which afflicts as many women as men.

After analyzing the blood of 13,000 people, scientists at the University of California in San Francisco, found that women with lower levels of vitamin C were more prone to gallbladder disease. Half of a papaya (about ten ounces) with 188mg magnesium and 150mg Vitamin C is needed in the diet and is a source of restoration of vitamin C. This exotic fruit can now be found in most supermarkets.

2. **Flaxseed.** Bakers use this nutty seed mainly to add flavor and fiber. But scientists see the tiny reddish seeds, rich in phytoestrogen compounds called lignans, as a potential weapon against breast cancer. A report mentioned in the symposium about breast cancer in San Antonio last year, showed that adding flaxseed to the diet of women with increasing breast cancer slowed the growth of the breast cancer tumor. You can flavor your muffins with flaxseed, but the easiest way to get the benefits is to sprinkle a few tablespoons of flaxseed on your cereal in the morning. Look for the seeds in natural food stores or supermarkets in the flour aisle. They are easy to grind in a grinder. But either way get the seeds – there aren't lignans in the oil.

3. **Tofu**. Foods high in soy protein can lower cholesterol and may minimize menopause and strengthen bones. Isoflavones, plant chemicals found in soybeans that have a structure similar to estrogen, may be the reason. Animal studies are, however, the bulk of the evidence, a human study found that 90mg of magnesium isoflavones was beneficial. And two other studies suggest that 50mg to 76mg of magnesium isoflavones a day may offer better maintenance to the heart and nervous system. ½ cup of tofu contains about 25mg to 35mg of magnesium isoflavones.

4. **Buffalo Meat**. Is good in large part to help menstruation, some women tend to be anemic more than men. And low iron levels in the blood can cause severe fatigue. To get a good dose of iron, try bison or buffalo, the meat is what women want- lots

of iron and less fat than most cuts of beef. "The iron content is about 3 mg per 3 ½ ounces in a raw portion. That same portion contains less than 3 grams of fat. Buffalo meat can help boost energy and lose weight. And you do not have to have a own a farm to get some bison. You can get it in many supermarkets.

5. **Chard**. This humble vegetable may help fight osteoporosis, which afflicts many women during their life. In addition to getting adequate amounts of calcium and vitamin D, there are some studies that suggest that vitamin K may also have a protective effect on bones. According to data from one of the largest studies, the study of health nurses, researchers found that women who ate more foods rich in vitamin K (at least 109 micrograms of the vitamin daily) were 30 percent less likely to suffer a hip fracture over ten years compared to women who ate less. The researchers point out that dark green leafy vehicles such as Brussel sprouts, spinach and broccoli are all good sources of the vitamin. But chard, with about 375 micrograms per half-cup, are among the better.

There you have it: five great foods for women and for men too whom both can stay healthy.

Antioxidants in vegetables;

The human body is composed of many different types of cells. Cells in turn are composed of different types of molecules.

Molecules consist of one or more atoms by complex electrochemical reactions. Over time cells of the human body begin to age.

The cells consist of many atoms. When they are healthy, the cells multiply and keep the body healthy and strong.

The quality of a healthy atom possesses "sandwiched electrons."

Antioxidant

An antioxidant is an atom that has an excess of electrons so it becomes the electron donor to the free radical, thus stopping the creation of a chained reaction of oxygenated radicals.

Antioxidant is a term that generally refers to a broad variety of vitamins, minerals and enzymes contained mostly in fruits and vegetables.

Numerous studies show that people who consume a good amount of fruits and vegetables are less likely to getting cancer, heart disease and generally do not have to do any kind of diet to maintain a healthy weight.

Some of the benefits of antioxidants for the body:

Prevent the formation of acne
Rejuvenate the skin
Increases the defensive power of the immune system
Helps the body to recover from the damage caused by excessive alcohol consumption.
Decreases allergic reactions
Protects against heart attacks
They keep arteries free of cholesterol
Relieve arthritis and muscle pain
Prevent intestinal inflammation
Prevents cancer development
Prevents hair loss
Prevents circulatory problems
Prevents colds and flu
Reduces fatigue
Helps in wound healing
Improves memory
Relieves symptoms of rheumatism
They energize the body
Reduce stress levels

The power of antioxidants is measured by their ability to absorb oxygen radicals, in a report by (USDA)

Plants with increased ability to reduce free radicals are:

	(Micrograms per 100.g):
Garlic. (Allium sativum):	.2000
Kale. (Brassica oleracea var acephala...):	.1770
Spinach. (Spinacia oleracea):	.1260
Alfalfa. (Medicago sativa) .sprouts:	.930
Broccoli. (Brassica italica oleracea.var...):	.890
Beet. (Beta vulgaris):	.840
Onion. (Allium cepa):	.450
Corn. (Zea mays):	.400
Eggplant. (Solanum melongena):.	.390
Pea. (Pisum sativum):	.390
Cabbage (Brassica capitata oleracea.var...).	.300
Potatoes. (Solana tuberosum):	.300
Lettuce. (Lactuca sativa):	.250
Carrot. (Daucus carota):	.200
Green Beans. (Phaseolus vulgaris):	.200
Tomatoes. (Lycopersicon esculentum):	.200
Celery. (Apium graveolens):	.100
Cucumber. (Cucumis sativus):	.100

Free Radicals

A free radical is an atom having at least one unpaired electron, i.e. it lacks one or more electrons. Radicals occur when oxygen is used to produce energy. Free radicals are created naturally by several biochemical processes involved in various functions of the body such as the metabolism, the body is able to control the number of radicals.

The problem occurs when excess radicals are present in the body for a long time. Sometimes and in some circumstances it could trigger a chain reaction of the production of free radicals, in a second one free radical may start a chain reaction and cause the production of one million or more free radicals. Free radicals alter or destroy cells. Cells that die and replicate in a defected state are cause of premature aging and all kinds of diseases.

Some of the conditions that favor creation of free radicals:

Physical exertion
Food additives
Pesticides
Pollution
Stress
Solar UV Radiation
Tobacco
Poor diet
Medication
Chlorine in water
Traveling on air planes
Dental fillings

Cinnamon and honey; are the only food substances on the planet that don't spoil or rot. Although its contents can be converted to sugars, honey is always honey.

If honey is left for long periods of time in a dark place it crystallizes. When this happens open the lid and heat with boiled water and let it melt. The honey will be as good new. Never boil honey or put it in the microwave, this will kill the enzymes. Cinnamon and honey can cure many diseases. (And the drug companies don't like this)

Honey is produced in most countries of the world. Science accepts honey as a very effective means of treating diseases.

Honey can be used without having any side effects and taken in the correct dose, even though it's sweet, it doesn't affect diabetics as much as artificial sweeteners, which do have side effects.

A list of diseases that can be cured by honey and cinnamon:

- Heart Disease

Make a paste of honey and cinnamon powder, apply it each morning to bread instead of jam and eat it regularly as part of breakfast. This will reduce the cholesterol in the arteries and saves the patient from having a heart attack. Also, those who have already had a heart attack, if they follow this process, will be protected from suffering another heart attack. Regular use of this concoction helps keep good smelling breathe, strengthens muscles and the rhythmic motion of the heart. In the United States and Canada, various nursing homes have successfully cured patients whose veins have lost their flexibility and have been plugged. Honey and cinnamon revitalized them.

- Arthritis

Arthritis patients may take every day, both in the morning and at night, a cup of hot water with two tablespoons of honey and one teaspoon of cinnamon powder. If taken regularly even chronic arthritis can be cured. Recent research done at the University of Copenhagen showed that doctors who treated their patients with a mixture of one tablespoon honey and 1/2 teaspoon cinnamon before breakfast, corroborated that in one week 73 out of 200 patients no longer felt arthritic pain, and after a month, almost all patients who could not walk or move because of pain, were moving without feeling pain.

- Digestion

Cinnamon sprinkled on two tablespoons of honey taken before meals can reduce acidity and to digest food more heavy.

- Cold and Flu

A scientist in Spain has proved that honey contains a natural ingredient which kills the influenza germ and protects patients from colds.

- Longevity

Tea made with honey and cinnamon powder, taken regularly reduces tissue damage caused by old age. Take four tablespoons of honey, one tablespoon of cinnamon powder and three cups of boiling water to make tea. Take a quarter cup, three to four times daily. It keeps the skin fresh and reduces the damage caused by the aging of tissues and free radicals, lengthening the period of regular vitality to over 100 years.

- Bladder Infections

Take two teaspoons of cinnamon powder and one tablespoon of honey in a glass of warm water and drink normally. It will destroy the germs in the bladder.

- Cholesterol

Two tablespoons honey and three teaspoons of cinnamon powder mixed with 16 ounces of tea administered to a patient with high levels of cholesterol, reduced cholesterol levels 10 percent in the first two hours of treatment. As mentioned earlier for arthritic patients, if taken three times a day, any chronic cholesterol disease is cured. According to information in this journal, pure honey taken as a daily food helps lower cholesterol.

- Colds

Those suffering from a severe head cold can take a spoonful of warm honey with 1/4 teaspoon cinnamon for three days. This process will cure any cold and clear the sinus.

- Stomach

Honey taken with cinnamon also helps heal the stomach, clears up and even heals ulcers completely.

- Gas

Studies in India and Japan revealed that honey and cinnamon reduce gas in the digestive system.

- Immune System

Daily use of honey and cinnamon powder strengthens the immune system and protects the body from bacteria and viruses. Scientists have found in honey various vitamins and iron in large amounts. Constantly using honey fortifies white blood cells and protects from diseases.

- Pimples

Three tablespoons of honey and cinnamon powder made into a paste, can be applied to pimples before going to bed, then washed the next day with warm water. If done for two weeks, pimples disappear even from the root.

- Skin Infections

Applying honey and cinnamon powder in equal parts to the affected area cure eczema and all types of skin infections.

- Weight Loss

In the morning, half an hour before breakfast and before going to sleep, drink a cup of boiled water with honey and cinnamon. If you drink regularly, it reduces the weight of even the most obese person. Also, drinking the mixture regularly does not allow the fat to accumulate in the body even if the person carries a high calorie diet.

- Cancer

Recent research in Japan and Australia have shown that advanced cancers of the stomach and bones have been totally cured. Patients suffering from these cancers should take one tablespoon of cinnamon and on of honey daily for a month three times a day.

- Fatigue

Studies have shown that the sugar content of honey is more helpful and does not weaken the amount of strength in the body. Senior patients who take honey and cinnamon powder in equal parts, are more alert and are more flexible. A cup of a tablespoon of honey and cinnamon powder daily upon rising and at 3 o'clock in the afternoon, when the vitality of the body starts to decrease, increases the vitality of the body in the space of just one week.

- Halitosis (Bad Breath)

People in South America occasionally gargle with a tablespoon of honey and cinnamon in hot water, keeping their breath fresh throughout day.

- Loss of Sense of Hearing

Honey and cinnamon taken in equal parts daily helps repair damaged tissue in the ear. Who does not remember as a child eating toast with butter and cinnamon?

If you wish to share this information with friends, loved ones and coworkers do it. We all need help and good health. What is done with the information in this book is the responsibility of everyone, recommending it as a book of daily family consultation.

20 tricks to befriend balance during pregnancy

One of the most common fears among pregnant women is getting fat during pregnancy and worse, keeping the extra pounds on after childbirth. To avoid the disturbance, and to women who do not want their weight to get out of control during the nine months pregnancy, first, it is crucial to forget the idea that you have to start eating for two as popular belief says about pregnancy. Increasing nine to 12 kilos (20-27lbs.) is normal, but above that level can be harmful to the mother and baby.

Nor should we abandon exercise. Simply adapt new routines to your new status, says Dr. Cury an orthopedist. According to the doctor, pregnant women can even lift weights, provided that it consists of light loads and under control preferably by a specialist. Ideally, though, are light exercises, not to lose muscle tone; and stretch a lot to maintain balance, as this will be a concern with the new weight of the belly, which puts pressure on the spine.

Here are 20 tips that experts recommend for moms to pass the nine months of pregnancy healthy and in good shape.

1. **Prefer small meals** every three hours, instead of a large lunch and dinner;
2. **To avoid morning sickness**, leave some dry foods (salty crackers, for example) next to your bed. Eat some before sitting up;
3. **Whole grains** are excellent sources of vitamin B complex, essential to minimize the discomfort of dizziness;
4. **Consume calcium** (dairy products), since it is a mineral that guarantees bone health for the mom;

5. **Do not forget the iron** (lean meats and vegetables) to prevent anemia;
6. **Include in your diet foods rich in folic acid**, which are in dark leaves, and ensures the formation of bone marrow in the baby;
7. **Eat a serving of grilled fish**, chicken or lean meat daily. In addition to the feeling of satiety, such foods generate enough protein for the baby and help the elasticity of the skin, preventing stretch marks;
8. **To avoid the feeling of being bloated**, very common in the last quarter, it is important to drink plenty of fluids and avoid excessive salt intake;
9. **The plate must be very colorful**, indicating a wide variety of nutrients;
10. **Prepare your meals calmly**, slowly swallowing food. This will facilitate digestion and prevent eating more than the appetite is actually asking for;
11. **Beware of diet foods** and excess sweeteners; these contain chemicals whose effects on your body should be discussed with your doctor;
12. **Avoid high fat foods**, such as milk and cream some types of red meat, cold cuts and sausages;
13. **Cut out the fried and breaded** for the nine months of gestation; they are only fattening foods, its nutrient content is not usable for you nor for the baby:
14. **When exercising**, try water aerobics, which is excellent for keeping in action all the muscles in your body without causing any impact which may compromise the baby;
15. **Stretch**; it helps to balance your body and prevents overloading of the spine;
16. **Lift weights**, but avoid high impact loads. During pregnancy, the important thing is to tone the muscles, and this is achieved with lighter sets, light weight and an instructor;
17. **Do not abuse** sweets and "cravings";
18. **Flee from** alcoholic drinks;

19. **Do not take weight loss medicines** (skinny pills) to moderate the appetite or metabolism boosters, which can cause damage the baby;
20. **If you feel heavy**, do not set your own diet, but diet under the guidance of a nutritionist.

Your Life: 10 ways to fight fat with fruit (1 of 8)

When you were young, your mother probably asked you to eat fruit. Although she was probably more interested in keeping you healthy -fruit has no cholesterol, it serves as a good source of heart healthy fiber and contains phytochemicals that reduce blood pressure and the risk of cancer and type 2 diabetes. Increasing your fruit intake may also help you lose weight. Add strawberries and grapefruit to your diet and watch the balance weight move inches to the left.

Your Life: 10 ways to fight fat with fruit (2 of 8)

Eat to lose weight

Research shows that listening to positive messages to lose weight or diets that promote eating more of certain foods provides better results than listening to negative messages or diets that promote eating less of certain foods. A recent study divided parents and children into two groups. The first group was given the positive message of eating more fruit, while the second group received a negative message eating less fat and sugar. The group that followed the positive message lost three times more weight during the study period.

Your Life: 10 ways to fight fat with fruit (3 of 8)

How to choose food

Everyone wants a weight loss plan that lets them eat as much as they wish and at the same time satisfy your hunger and reduce calorie intake. The trick is to choose foods with a lower energy density, or fewer calories per gram of food. The larger the amount of water and fiber in a food, the lower the energy density it provides. That will help you stay full and at the same time, reduce your caloric intake and make the weight go down.

Your Life: 10 ways to fight fat with fruit (4 of 8)

Fruit . . . But not just any fruit!

One of the best ways to stock up with low energy density food is to eat more fruit. But not just any fruit. Canned fruit in heavy syrup has twice the energy density of canned fruit with light syrup. Nuts have four times the energy density than fresh fruit because almost all the water has been removed. The best option for fewer calories and to get the feeling of fullness and satisfaction is fresh whole fruit. The main fruits for weight loss include grapefruit, melons (watermelon and honeydew) (strawberries, raspberries and blueberries), papaya and peach.

Your Life: 10 ways to fight fat with fruit (5 of 8)

10 easy tricks to increase your intake of fruit

According to mypyramid.gov, women should eat at least two cups of fruit per day and if you are physically active you should consume even more. Here are some suggestions to help increase your fruit intake to healthier levels . . . and can help to shed off a few pounds in the process.

1) **In a restaurant.**
    Of course you would like to order a cheesecake for dessert, however, consider the following option. Many restaurants serve plates of fruit accompanied by a tasty indulgence of a sugar cookie, a scoop of sorbet or a selection cheese.

2) **Apples anytime.**
   Eat apple slices in abundance throughout the day. This way the temptation to buy sweets out of the vending machine will be lower.

3) **Do your cravings for ice cream late at night ruin your diet?**
   Instead of ice cream, eat frozen grapes. They are sweet, crunchy and cold - and they will make you forget about the ice cream in your freezer.

4) **Fruit or fried**. More than just a couple letters of difference. When eating at fast food chains, ask for a cup of fruit instead of fried food.

5) **Surprise with fruit**.
   Donuts and muffins can be your usual breakfast on your way to work. But try it and surprise your colleagues with a dessert of frozen berries, yogurt and low fat granola.

6) **As a companion.**
   If you usually eat fries with your lunch sandwich, try replacing them with a grapefruit. Peel and cut the grapefruit in the morning before going to work and put it in a re-sealable plastic bag.

7) **With cereals.**
   Liven up your breakfast with a handful of berries in your cold cereal or adding sliced peaches to oatmeal.

8) **A tasty and quick dish for dinner**
   Try this dessert with fruit. Slice strawberries and mix with raspberries and blueberries. Cover with syrup. To make the syrup: simmer ½ cup of water with 2 tablespoons dark brown sugar until reduced to 1/4 cup. Let it cool and pour over fruit for an out of this world dessert.

9) **Fruit as an appetizer.**
Finger foods can ruin your diet because they have a lot of calories and fat. Surprise your friends with a delicious appetizer, low in calories and colorful fruit kebab. Cut up different fruits and put them on a bamboo stick. Some fruits that can be used are red and green grapes, pieces of pineapple, strawberries, sliced bananas, pear cubes . . . the sky is the limit! If you prepare in advance, moistened the fruit with lemon juice to prevent the bananas and pears from turning brown or oxidizing.

10) **Fruits always at your fingertips.**
Have a bowl of fresh fruit on your kitchen counter. You will be more likely to eat an apple, a tangerine or peach if they are visible.

Now we'll tell you how to meet the nutritional needs of your teenage children.

Organizing a teenager's diet. . . Mission impossible?

Teens have important nutritional needs. . . What should a parent do?

A hallmark of adolescence is to grow autonomy and independence of the family and parents, and teens are more inclined to eat away from home than ever before. But teenagers have important nutritional needs. So, what's a parent to do?

The facts:

1. **Increased independence**
Teenagers often eat with friends rather than with the family. They have more control over their food choices, often practice fad diets, adopt new tendencies and consume various types of food.

2. **What interests them**
    Most teenagers are more concerned with achieving athletic
    prowess and in their image than in protecting their long-term
    health. They tend to limit the consumption of calories and fats
    to lose weight and downplay the importance of maintaining a
    healthy cardiovascular system.

    Adolescent athletes are also susceptible to the use of ergogenic
    supplements which often are not tested and can have serious
    side effects.

3. **Nutritional needs**
    The vital nutrients during adolescence are iron, calcium and
    total calorie intake. Studies on the diets of teens show they
    often lack sufficient amounts of iron and calcium which will
    enhance their growth and health. If teens limit calorie intake to
    manage body weight, growth can really be affected negatively.

What to do?

Most of the foundation of the diet for your teenager rests with the
meals and snacks you provided them in their early life. However,
there are some important things you can do to continue to
positively influence their diet:

-   Give them structured meals and ensure that your child eat
    with the family at least once a day. This will provide both the
    opportunity to include healthy foods in their diet and talk
    about their day and their experiences.
-   Make sure your home has a good stock of healthy snacks. Keep
    fruit, breads, bagels, juices, cheese sticks and yogurt, within
    reach and readily available.
-   Talk to your teens about their options when at lunch.
    Encourage them to drink orange juice instead of sodas, and
    consider adding fruit or vegetables in their lunches. Find out
    what meals and snacks are available at their school.

- Avoid criticizing the food choices of your teen. When food becomes a topic of discussion, studies show that adolescents avoid more meals and opt for worse food. Despite the fears of parents, most teens somehow overcome these difficult years. Unless you notice your child is losing more weight than is healthy, or looks like he is relying on supplements rather than whole foods, stay out of the way and let them experiment.

Health - Very Important Tips

Answer the phone with LEFT ear
Do not drink coffee.
Do not take pills with COOL water

Do not eat heavy meals after 5pm. Reduce the amount of OIL in the foods you eat. Drink more WATER in the morning, less at night. Keep your distance from wireless phone chargers, home or cellphones. Do not use wireless phones or headsets for a LONG period of time. The best time to sleep is 10 pm at night to 6am in the morning. Do not lie down immediately after taking medicine before sleeping. When the battery is low, on the LAST bar, do not answer the phone, radiation is 1000 times greater.

Here are some tips for maintaining physical and mental health.

"An ounce of prevention is better than pound of cure"

Healthy Juices

Carrot + Ginger + Apple - Boosts and cleans our system.

Apple + Cucumber + Celery - Prevents cancer, reduces cholesterol and stomach problems and eliminates headaches.

Tomato + Carrot + Apple - Improves skin appearance and eliminates bad breath.

Bitter pumpkin + Apple + Milk - Avoids bad breath and reduces internal body heat.

Pineapple + Apple + Watermelon – Dispels excess salts, nourishes the kidneys and bladder.

Orange + Ginger + Cucumber - Improves the texture and moisture of the skin and reduces body heat.

Apple + Cucumber + Kiwi - Improves skin complexion.

Pear & Banana - regulates sugar content.

Carrot + Apple + Pear + Mango - Regulates body heat, counteracts toxicity, decreases blood pressure and fights against oxidation.

Melon + Grape + Watermelon + Milk - Rich in vitamin C + Vitamin B2 which increases cell activity and strengthens body immunity.

Papaya + Pineapple + Milk - Rich in vitamin C, E and iron. Improves flexibility of the skin and metabolism.

Banana + Pineapple + Milk - Rich in vitamins and nutrients that prevent colds.

Pretty interesting! AUTO Shiatsu

Just, look at this. . . .

The organs of your body have sensory points on the soles of your feet. If you massage these points you will find relief from aches and pains. As you can see, the heart is on the left foot.

Shown as points and arrows to show which organ connects where.

It is indeed correct since the nerves connected to these organs end here.

This is seen in great detail by studies of acupressure and textbooks.

God created our body so well that he thought of this. He made us walk so that we will always be pressing these pressure points and therefore maintain these organs, activating them at all times.

Keep walking. . . .

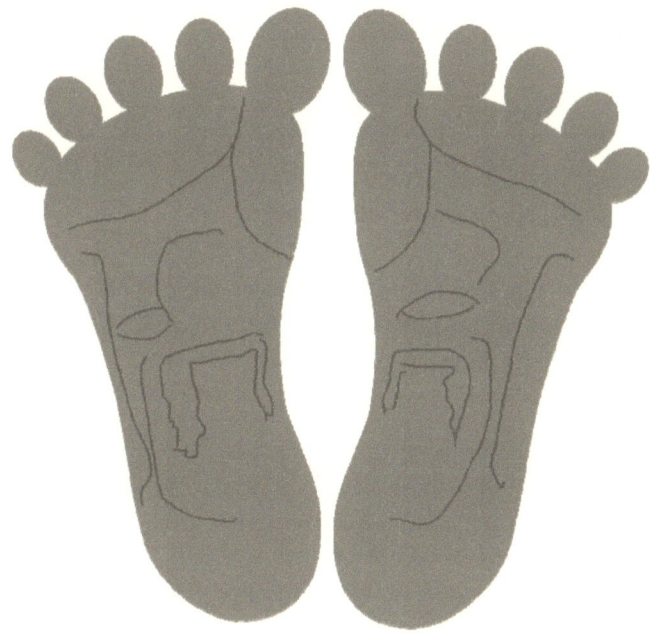

Did you know your blood type reveals your personality?

Type Of Blood And RH Factor	# Of People Who Have It
O+	40%
O -	7%
A +	34%
A -	6%
B +	8%
B -	1%
AB +	3%
AB-	1%

Your blood type reveals your personality?

According to a Japanese institute that does research on blood types, there are certain personality traits that seem to coincide with certain blood types. How do you value yourself?

Type O	You want to become a leader and when you see something you want you strive to achieve your goal. You are a trendsetter, loyal, passionate, and have confidence in yourself. Your weaknesses include vanity and jealousy and you tend to be too competitive.
Type A	You like harmony, peace and organization. You work well with others, you are sensitive, patient and affectionate. Your weaknesses are your stubbornness and inability to relax

Type B	You're a rugged individualist looking forward and like to do things your way. Creative and flexible, you adapt easily to any situation. But your insistence to stay independent can sometimes go too far and become a weakness.
Type AB	Cool and collected, you are generally a good person and read people easily. You are a natural artist because of your tact and you're fair. But you are confrontational, blunt and it's hard for you to make decisions.

	You can receive blood from:							
If your blood type is:	O-	O+	B-	B+	A-	A+	AB-	AB+
AB+	Y	Y	Y	Y	Y	Y	Y	Y
AB-	Y		Y		Y	Y		
A+	Y	Y			Y	Y		
A-	Y				Y			
B+	Y	Y	Y	Y				
B-	Y		Y					
O+	Y	Y						
O-	Y							

KNOW ABOUT THE BENEFITS OF CONSUMING FRUITS AND VEGETABLES

Fruit	Benefit	Benefit	Benefit	Benefit	Benefit
Apple	Protects the heart	Prevents Constipation	Stops diarrhea	Helps lung capacity	betters arteries
Apricot	Combats Cancer	Controls blood pressure	Saves your sight	Fights Alzheimer's	Slows down aging process
Artichoke	Helps digestion	Reduces cholesterol	Protects the heart	Stabilizes blood sugar	Protects against liver disease
Avocado	Combats diabetes	Reduces cholesterol	Helps detain cerebral vascular accidents	Controls blood pressure	Smoothes skin
Banana	Protects the heart	Weakens cough	fortifies your bones	Controls blood pressure	Detains Diarrhea
Beans	Prevents constipation	helps with hemorrhoids	Reduces Cholesterol	Combats Cancer	Stabilizes blood sugar
Beets	Controls blood pressure	Combats Cancer	fortifies your bones	Protects the heart	Helps to lose weight
Blueberry	Combats Cancer	Protects the heart	Stabilizes blood sugar	Helps Memory	Prevents Constipation
Broccoli	Fortifies your bones	Saves sight	combats cancer	Protects the heart	Controls blood pressure
Cabbage	Combats Cancer	Prevents Constipation	Promotes weight loss	Protects the heart	Helps control hemorrhoids
Cantaloupe	Saves sight	Controls blood pressure	Reduces Cholesterol	Combats Cancer	Supports the Immune System

DRINK WATER WHEN YOU WAKE UP

It is popular in Japan today to drink water immediately after waking up every morning. Furthermore, scientific tests have proven its worth. We publish below a description of the use of water for our readers. For old and serious diseases as well as modern illnesses, water treatment has been found to be successful by a Japanese medical society as a 100% cure for the following diseases:

Headache, body ache, heart system, rapid heartbeat, arthritis, epilepsy, excess weight, bronchitis, asthma, TB, meningitis, kidney and urine diseases, vomiting, gastritis, diarrhea, diabetes, constipation, all eye diseases, womb, cancer and menstrual disorders, diseases of the ear, nose and throat.

METHOD OF TREATMENT

1. When you wake up in the morning before brushing your teeth, drink 4 x 160ml glasses of water. . . . Interesting
2. Brush and clean the mouth but do not eat or drink anything for 45 minutes.
3. After 45 minutes you may eat and drink normal.
4. After 15 minutes of eating breakfast, lunch and dinner, don't eat or drink anything for 2 hours.
5. Those who are too old or sick and cannot drink 4 glasses of water at the beginning may commence by taking little water and gradually increase up to 4 glasses per day.
6. The above method of treatment will cure diseases of the sick and others can enjoy a healthy life.

The following list indicates the number of days of treatment required to cure, control and reduce the main diseases:

1. Gastric - 10 days
2. Constipation - 10 days
3. Diabetes - 30 days

4. High Blood Pressure - 30 days
5. TB - 90 days
6. Cancer - 180 days
7. Arthritis patients should follow the above treatment only for 3 days the 1st week, and every day of the 2nd week and onwards.

This treatment method has no side effects, nonetheless at the beginning of treatment you may need to urinate several times.

It is better if we continue this and make this treatment as a routine in our life.

Drink water and stay healthy and active.

This makes sense. The Chinese and Japanese drink hot tea with their meals. Not cold water. Maybe it is time we adopt their habit of drinking while eating. Nothing to lose, everything to gain . . . for those who like to drink cold water, this article is applies to you.

It is common to have a cold drink after a meal. However, the cold water will solidify the oily stuff that you have just ingested.

This slows digestion and hardens more fat in your body.

Once this "sludge" reacts with the acid, it will decompose and will be absorbed faster in the intestine than solid foods.

It will line the intestine. Soon, it will become fats and can lead to cancer. It is best to drink hot soup or warm water after a meal.

A serious note about heart attacks: Women should know that not every heart attack symptoms will be in the left arm:

You may never have the first chest pain during the course of a heart attack. Nausea and intense sweating are also common symptoms.

60% of people who have a heart attack while they are asleep do not wake up.

Be aware of intense pain in the jaw line. Pain in the jaw can wake you from a sound sleep. Let's be careful and be aware. The more we know, the better the opportunity for us to survive. . .

Seven things you should not do after a meal

Do not smoke after a meal! Expert experimented and found that smoking a cigarette after a meal is comparable to smoking TEN cigarettes (chances of cancer is higher).

Do not eat fruits immediately after meals. The stomach will swell and bloat. Therefore, eat your fruits half an hour before or two hours after a meal.

Do not tighten your belt after eating. Tightening the belt after a meal can cause intestinal problems.

Do not bathe after eating. Bathing increases the blood flow to the hands, legs and body thereby causing the amount of blood around the stomach to decrease. This will weaken the digestive system of our stomach.

Do not walk after eating even when you have heard people say to walk a hundred steps after a meal and you will live till 99. Walking immediately after a meal would hinder the digestive system to absorb the nutrition from the food eaten. Wait at least one hour after a meal and then walk if you want to.

Do not sleep immediately after eating. Food may not be digested properly and this causes gastro-intestinal problems.

Do not make love immediately after a meal because it can be extremely dangerous. This is cause for much discussion, because the experts do not agree. Yes it is confirmed, it can interrupt digestion and you can have a heart attack, especially those with coronary problems.

Do not read after eating this may put more strain on the body. Do not work on the computer or read the newspaper while eating. Do not drive or work while eating breakfast or lunch. . . even though these things are not checked by doctors, eventually it will affect your metabolism. . . enjoy one of the major pleasures of life. . . eating. . . eating while sitting at the table or at a picnic, enjoying nature or enjoying the company of our family or partner is most sacred and we have to take care of this. . .

In big cities with a lot of hustle and stress, in most jobs, you only get 30 minutes for lunch where many have to go to fast food places and run to work while others are eating while driving to make it back to their shift . . . although there is not an actual statistic we can see that the results are very obvious . . . today we have more problems of obesity, colon problems, diabetes and more deaths from heart disease than ever before.

Conclusion . . . need more proof?

In other Latin American and European countries midday break hours for employee are two hours which allows those who live nearby their home to eat there or take the time to eat and have normal digestion. . .

(1) D & C: 89 shall run and not be weary; and shall walk and not faint (Doctrine and covenants LDS TRIPLE) there is a promise in the word of wisdom and health. . . it is one of the few principles with a promise. . . yes, it says that they will run and not be weary and they shall walk and not faint, and how many of us have climbed three stair cases and we're tired, we walk a block and it seems as though we'll already pass out. . . even though it sounds exaggerated, fatigue exists in our body which isn't normal and we blame it on age; "it's because we're getting

old," without wanting to acknowledge that we have abused our temple. . . we say don't smoke or drink coffee and in that we are fulfilling the word of wisdom. . . but we still haven't fulfilled that which will allow us to "run and not be weary and walk and not faint."

(2) Genesis 1:29-30 (what was told to Adam and Eve???) Every green herb will be for food. Since Adam and Eve we were told to eat plants and fruit for meat . . . not all kinds of canned and artificial flavors and colors . . .for this reason people in the past lasted longer and we will also add that there was not much contamination. . . they lived long and healthy for many years but not sick. . . without pains. . .

(3) Moses also was given a revelation of health which gives a list of more specific instructions about what to eat and what not to eat . . . which was more than just a simple commandment of obligation but truly wise instructions of how to live more healthy and care for the temple of God which you yourselves are. . . it said that certain animals such as pigs should not be eaten because they were contaminated. . . of course many took it as a spiritual obligation not realizing that God was saving their mortal life. . . Pork in itself contains a poisonous contaminant parasite and is explosive to the body of a human being which does not affect pigs. . . it is a parasite called (Trichinella spiralis) which are poisonous eggs that go to the brain. Which flames can't even kill it, but can only be at low freezing temperatures for long periods of time up to 90 days. . .Trichinellosis is an infectious disease caused by various species of the genus Trichinella parasite especially Trichinella spiralis. This disease is also known as the Trichinellosis. Even though in the United States they have a higher degree of caution when preparing pork one must still be careful when eating it.

The disease is acquired as a result of ingestion of red or undercooked meat of animals infected with cysts that contain the larvae of the parasite. This infection is common in carnivore animals such as bear, fox, or lion, but can also exist in rats, horses, wild boars and domestic animals like the pig. Encapsulated larvae can survive years in the muscle tissue of the host. The ingestion of pork is what infects men most with the infection. The geographical distribution is worldwide and is still common in parts of Europe and the United Sates. The population at risk are consumers of meat products from hunts and domestic kills. How is the disease produced? After consuming infected meat with Trichinella Spiralis cysts, stomach acid can dissolve the capsule covering the parasite releasing the worms inside. The worms reproduce and pass through the intestinal wall into the bloodstream. Through the arteries, they are transported to the muscles and invade them, and there they can encyst again. These organisms tend to invade muscle tissues, including the heart and diaphragm and even reach the lungs and brain. This infection is not spread from person to person and the only way to acquire it is eating meat that contains this live parasite.

Fish is one of the best sources of animal protein you can get, with the advantage of no saturated fats and you do get omega 3 and 6 which are beneficial to your cardiovascular system.

In fact, people who eat fish twice a week, reduce, by 30%, the chance of heart disease.

Properties:

- Contains high levels of vitamin A, D and B
- Prevents oxidation
- It has Omega 3 acids which prevent heart disease and helps lower cholesterol
- It is easy to prepare
- Contains no saturated fat

The Bad

Some species are contaminated with mercury, a substance that can cause brain damage. Furthermore, due to contamination of some sea fish, it is believed that certain species may have a substance linked to cancer: polychlorinated biofenil. (ESPECIALLY SCALELESS FISH BECAUSE THEY ARE THE FISH THAT REMAIN NEAR THE SHORE EATING LARVAE AND CONTAMINATION. . .)

The best counsel, in this case, is to eat fish 2 times a week, but be careful that it is not of the same species, as this will make sure you're getting all the necessary nutrients and not consuming harmful substances in excess.

Avoid species that are considered "highly contaminated" such as shark, catfish and swordfish; and eat preferably tuna, salmon, and merganser, crappie, croaker, in the end fish with scales and fins.

Why not shark or catfish? Or why should fish without scales not be eaten according to the Law of Moses? Note that the scales of fish help fish to withstand the water pressure and can therefore reach deep depths of the ocean and can feed on seaweed, plants and species of the sea. . . On the other hand, catfish are only in the banks and feed on larvae and garbage and the same with sharks, where they have found metal license plates inside their stomachs and even eat human beings, and Catfish are the pigs of the sea. . .(eat all kinds of garbage).

For some reason God gave these instructions to Moses, who most benefit from this is us. It is not mentioned in any part of the Bible that they were punished for not following this law, it only mentioned that they would be contaminated and deprived of the privilege to enter the temple and given a few days to decontaminate yourself and that if anyone destroys their temple, which is us, that God would destroy us; but it didn't mean that he would strike us with a lightning rod or something like that but simply that we destroy ourselves by intoxicating and contaminating ourselves, without the right to demand blessings of health. . .

All these animals mentioned in the Law of Moses are related with sicknesses and some diseases that are produced in the body . . . verified by real doctors and naturopathic doctors and also nutritionists. . .

(5) Also in 1833 modern health revelations were given . . . where Joseph Smith being a man with only a third grade education . . . gives health instructions received from God that match the New Food Pyramid. . .

D&C 89

Every herb in the season thereof, and every fruit in the season thereof... flesh also of beasts for the use of man . . .(however it must be used **limitedly**.) And it is pleasing unto me that they should not be used, only in times of winter, or of cold, or famine.

18. And all saints who remember to keep and do these sayings, walking in obedience to the commandments, shall receive health in their navel and marrow to their bones.

The word of wisdom doesn't tell us exactly what we should avoid or consume, but it gives us guidelines. (Gospel Principles Pg. 187)

PH Balance (Potential Hydrogen)

In 1909, a Danish biochemist named; Soren Peter L. discovered that all diseases are based on one thing; in the self-intoxication of the body.

He found that all health or sickness depends on the balance of the body called PH. (potential hydrogen)

It consists of that if your body is acidic you're sick and if your body is alkaline you are healthy.

It's quite simple, the majority of the most delicious or popular fast foods are the most damaging to convert your body acidic. Some of the characteristics of the acidity of the body is due to; foods with excess oil (fried), white flour without fiber which makes the body receive more glucose and activates the pancreas creating a madness of excess sugars. . .The famous energy drink. . . caffeine, soda, hot dogs; if we only knew how hot dogs are made we would never eat any more of them. They grind all the remains and leftovers of the slaughter house, once ground they add in the same flavor and the same coloring so that everything looks and tastes like one flesh. . .

And all these things like; alcohol, coffee, Gatorade, chips, energy drinks, etc. gradually deteriorate the body until it is degraded and becomes prematurely old. Studies on PH indicate that in an alkaline body does disease cannot exist. And what makes a body alkaline? Greens, vegetables and fruits. Nutritionists recommend that for a body to be completely healthy it requires 6 fruits and 4 vegetables daily and that's where the Drubinlife mix comes from. Because who eats 4 vegetables and at least 6 fruits daily???? Hardly anyone, right? For that reason this green smoothie works. . .

And if accompanied by exercise it will be even more effective

(8)   Also, in an alkaline environment exists vegetation and life. In an acidic environment everything dries up and dies . . . and thus like this our cells slowly do the same thing inside us. . . in an alkaline fish tank the fish are happy, but in an acidic fish tank the fish die. This happens to so many people and they don't know the reason why. If you do not control the pH of your aquarium the fish die and the same happens with your own body, it deteriorates rapidly. . .

(9)   **When water was water** . . . now it has all of this: arsenic, microbes, lead, pesticides . . . and when the air was air people lasted longer . . . and now we are speeding up global warming . . . the ozone layer is going . . . and our air is more

polluted . . . when the food was organic . . . now we eat more pesticides and chemicals. . .

(10) An acid body is always going to be sick, and an alkaline body is always going to be healthy. . .

(11) Let's compare our body with carnivores or herbivores

Starting with this carnivorous animal; The Tiger!

Note that it has fangs for tearing flesh, has claws to tear its prey, it doesn't have molars and does not chew food, its intestine is as short as less than a half meter; whatever it eats its stomach digests it quickly, like that of a dog. The intestine of a human being is 18 meters and we have molars. A cow's is 46 meters and also has molars and even four stomachs, no fangs or claws and feed only on green pastures, do not suffer from diabetes and chew their food well. . .

(12) What are we then? Omnivores (pig)? Let's compare ourselves to an omnivore. What do omnivores eat? All kinds of garbage . . . are we sometimes like the omnivores . . .?

(13) Ghoulish as the Vulture? . . . What do ghouls eat? Carrion (dead) sometimes we resemble Ghouls . . . eating excessive meat. . .

(14) We have become chemicalvores . . . a chemicalvore is one that feeds on pure chemical sweetened-dyes. . . (Poisonous dyes, medications, preservatives, artificial flavors . . . sweetened-dyes . . . chemical sugar and Yellow # 3 # 5 the same dye used for disinfectants and liquid bathroom cleaners.

(15) What are we then really? We are herbivores . . . human beings are phytophagous, because we were designed to live healthier with fruits, seeds and vegetables. . .

(16) Have you ever seen an aesthetic tiger? Or a rabbit with glasses? Or diabetic cow?

(17) FOOD FOR THE PANCREAS; what is the function of the pancreas? The pancreas is located between the liver and the stomach, the function of the pancreas is to control the glucose of the body. It creates and sends the insulin that the body needs to help to form the cells, close wounds and sustain life. . .

What does the pancreas feed on? Only green vegetables . . . we can eat everything at a buffet but if we do not eat anything green it doesn't do any good, the pancreas has not been fed. . . and what happens when a pancreas is not fed? It dies of hunger and a dead pancreas is a diabetic and a diabetic is a dead pancreas.

I emphasize, again, the only thing that feeds the pancreas are greens (green plants) and the more the better.

(18) THE NUMBER ONE ENEMY TO HEALTH IS CONSTIPATION. . .

All diseases depend on this organ, all are concentrated there because of poor diet and little fiber intake in the body;

And if food is low in fiber and worse when meat is added it remains trapped which creates a lethal condition for the body. . .

Those 18 meters of intestines are doing all the work distributing vitamins, enzymes, minerals, and amino acids. . . what goes in must come out in 24-34 hours if not, this causes a problem for the body because what the body does not need should be disposed of in these 24 hours and if you eat three times a day you should go to the bathroom 3 times daily. . . otherwise the putrefaction remains and cannot be disposed of the body.

The walls of the intestines are lined with membranes that resemble a broccoli top. These are what allow the absorption of nutrients and distribute all that the body needs. Soda, especially, contains an acid that closes these membranes and does not allow its proper function. . . Imagine putting oils, fats and white flour in the washer, it won't be long before it is plugged.

(19) From here, then, the colon deteriorates. If we destroy our colon, wecould do a colostomy operation which means they

cut meters off the intestine or colon and you will not be able to defecate normal. . .

These organs do not regenerate unless you change your diet. . .

(21) THE EVOLUTION OF HEALTH:

What have we done with our health? When we were small we ate jams, fruits, soups . . . as we grow we change our diets and begin to tell mom; I want a pizza! Sitting in front of a TV playing a game. . . Also, if we go out we just say "take us to the burger joint". . . (Fast Food) . . . therefore many kids will ask, "What are we going to eat?" because they have always eaten the same as the food. . . Here I will show you how to start.

CARBONATION VS WATER. . .

Many people think that because they do not drink coffee they have achieved are fulfilling the word of wisdom because nowhere Pepsi or Coke appears as part of the word of wisdom . . . without knowing it is even worse, because soda contains 34 milligrams of caffeine (water soluble) and is equivalent to more than ten cups of coffee. Caffeine is added to create an addiction and dependence for people, also, the amount of sugar it has creates dependency.

Amount of caffeine per cup of instant coffee:

Decaffeinated coffee one cup 2 mg
Special coffee 16 to 18 mg
Strong coffee 80 mg
Instant Coffee 120 mg

What's more, the sugars contained in soda, gradually dissolve tooth enamel, weakening teeth and producing cavities. Not only that, the sugars that the body is unable to digest, become fat, leading to the possible consequence of being overweight and even obesity.

Previously diabetes was associated with adult patients, but in recent times we have seen an increase in cases of this disease in children and adolescents who are overweight. There are currently 22 million children under 5 years old who are overweight and have diabetes. Diabetes is a disease that affects mainly the eyes, bones, kidneys, feet and heart. And recently it has been discovered that there are more ingredients that produce cancer.

YOU NEED APPROXIMATELY 32 GLASSES OF WATER TO PURIFY YOURSELF OF ONE SODA AND TO DETOXIFY YOUR BLOOD OF THIS SLOW DEATH POISON. . .

A caffeinated diet like tea, coffee, soda pop and chocolate drinks is not good for you. In some studies done in New York in recent years, volunteers were studied for 6 years and in this period 349,282 died of a heart attack and 67 of a stroke. The American expert emphasized that the effects of caffeine are usually seen after the age of 65. He found that those who drink caffeinated drinks their whole lives no longer have the same protection after about 65 years of age than they did when they were younger and that's when the illnesses begin to happen. In some cases, it happens when they're younger than 65.

Coffee and tea, chocolate and cola drinks contain, besides caffeine, compounds such as phosphoric acid and carbonation or other ingredients that might be adulterated. Notice in the table below the amounts of caffeine that are added to these drinks to create dependence. . .

Although there are many contradictions that say coffee helps reduce the risk of heart attacks, on the flip side, it produces an increase in blood pressure . . . nothing is guaranteed, and moreover the doctors or medical students never agree on the subject which on one side it supposedly helps you and on the other side it hurts you . . .

They say it takes away headaches while on the other side it becomes a drug that one becomes dependent upon and if they don't drink coffee it gives them a headache (sound familiar?) Like drugs that make you dependent . . . these effects are not immediate but usually occur after 60 years old and in some cases many years before, between 40 and 50 years. . .

The Prophet Joseph Smith claims to have received a revelation on 27 February 1833 in Ohio D&C 89: 9 And again, hot drinks are not for the body or belly.. . . in modern revelations current church leaders say that this refers to coffee (caffeinated or decaffeinated it's the same) and tea . . . especially those that are not natural and that come in little bags that you boil. . .

Today soda has become very popular and has created dependency for that reason those who think "I do not drink coffee", but drink more soda daily than water are even more at risk because of the amount of added caffeine and high glucose that the body does not need. Also, we add carbon acids which are not vitamins. And even diet sodas (diet coke) are harmful for a weak body which are scarce in vitamins and have poor nutrition. . .

energy drinf

The propaganda and its slogan says; THE ONLY BULL THAT GIVES YOU WINGS . . . yeah, to fly to heaven. . .

Energy Drinks was created to stimulate the brains in people subjected to great physical exertion and in a "stress coma" and never be consumed like an innocent refreshing drink. France and Denmark have prohibited it as a cocktail of death, due to components of mixtures "GLUCURONOLACTONE" a highly dangerous chemical for the organism, was discontinued in several European countries due to the high index of cases of migraines, cerebral tumors and liver disease and cause of cardiac arrest. . .

Energy drinks are considered to be highly dangerous drinks . . . they up your energy, apparently the way it works is that it dissolves the blood so that the heart gives less effort . . . and the energy it gives you is an artificial, temporary energy, and then comes a fall or downturn in mood. . .

It directly alters the central nervous system, increases resistance and delays the onset of tiredness. It affects cardiovascular functions, heart rate and blood pressure. This causes extra systoles, palpitations, increased blood pressure, fast pulse and angina-like chest pain. And it was used as an anticoagulant and to do dialysis for patients with chronic renal illness so the blood does not clot.

A little like sodium heparin (anticoagulant) drug which is used for chronic kidney patients which dialysis is performed. So that the blood doesn't clot and they can do the treatment on a machine for about 3-4 hours maximum in a span of 3 sessions per week

Taurine (bull accelerator) Also known as 2-aminoethanesulfonic acid, taurine was originally isolated from bull bile in 1827 in Germany. At the present time it's produced synthetically and is the magic elixir that will give us energy. Taurine effects are powerful, even contained in a single tin: Not only an inhibitory neurotransmitter (acting in some cases, as a sedative, anticoagulant), and an antioxidant that defies age; it also has the potential to regulate tachycardia.

80mg Caffeine

Ah, here are the wings of **Energy Drinks**- 80mg to 120mg of caffeine. Here are all the things this drink should presumably do for us – increase our concentration and reaction speed, improve emotional state, and boost metabolism – these are all known effects of this white powder, a distant cousin of cocaine.

Inositol (B complex)

It also contains a carbohydrate found in animal muscle (sometimes called "meat sugar"), inositol which is becoming a magic drug that significantly reduces depression, seizures, panic attacks, agoraphobia, and obsessive-compulsive disorder. Instead of being one of the ingredients in **Energy Drinks**, inositol should really be a drink by itself.

It is a carbonated beverage containing primarily water, sugar (saccharin, glucose), taurine, glucuronolactone and caffeine, as well as different vitamins (niacin, pathogenic acid, B6 and B12). According to the manufacturer, it has an energizing and detoxifying effect, also, properties that increase physical capabilities and speeds up the mind etc. Causing euphoria and increased heart rate, this animal liver protein in energy drinks containing caffeine, taurine and other compounds that stimulate concentration and physical endurance have become fashionable in the streets, offices, parties and sports.

"Red Bull", "Rockstar," "Monster," "Roaring Lion", "Rush", "Go Fast" or "Dark Dog" appeal to younger people and have become the fastest growing segment in the non-alcoholic beverage market of The United States, according to several studies.

All are carbonated and served cold, they are generally lemon flavored, containing one or more stimulants mainly caffeine, guarana and taurine.

The most popular brand is "**Energy Drinks**," which is "designed for periods of mental and physical stress" and "can be drunk in virtually any situation while you practice a sport, driving, at work or in recreation."

"**Energy Drinks**" contains 80 milligrams of caffeine, a stimulant that raises adrenaline levels and alertness, and 1,000 milligrams of taurine, an amino acid that helps in the function of the heart and the brain.

Although medical studies on energy drinks are still scarce, this brand has already been banned in some countries due to concerns of the effects of ingesting taurine in high doses would have on health.

*** It has also sparked controversy over mixing it with alcohol, a particularly striking fashion at parties and bars, and among those under 30 years old, the consumer profile to which the products are intended. ***

"Energy drinks are not a healthy practice or solution. We need to increase our energy naturally, keeping a healthy diet and exercising regularly," drinking Drubin-life daily.

Since the release of "Red Bull" in 1997, there have been 200 other brands emerge, and with them a number of trends and categories, such as those involving aphrodisiacs, diet or sugar free, nutritional and for the more seasoned, the 500 milliliter drinks.

Water, Sugar (saccharin, glucose), taurine, glucuronolactone and caffeine, and various vitamins (niacin, pantothenic acid, B6 and B12).

Some experts agree that the risk of energy drinks is its mixture with other substances, in particular, with alcohol and coffee: mixing stimulants with depressants can cause abnormal heart rhythms, and can create problems in the future.

Taurine and caffeine. . . The key here is mixing these two together produces what is called "mortal energy reaction."

OBECITY PROBLEMS

We can see the reality of this famous logo

Sodas dark drinks carbonated

This child is 5 years old and many people think they have to sue fat food's, who should be sued are the parents. . .

FAST FOOD;

One of the ironies is the commercials always make it look very attractive, makes you look slim and beautiful and keep a good figure, when it is not true. All these ads show beautiful bodies but the reality is different. . . excess sugars contained in these drinks and the amount of fat found in "fast foods" which if you just take the S out of fast it means it will fatten you "FAT FOOD" which is only a sickness waiting to happen and early death for the future of these new generations.

WHAT SHOULD WE EAT?

That's the question we all ask ourselves. . .

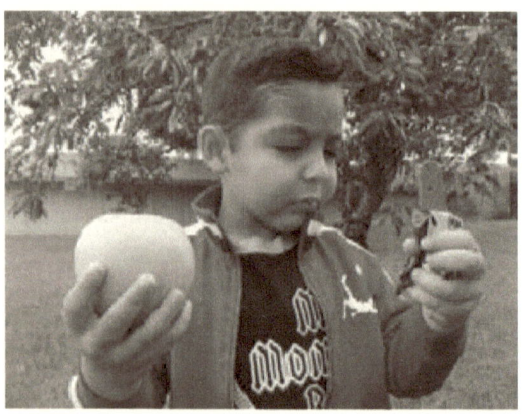

The first problem is that we let our children choose between sweets or natural fruit. . . what do you believe the child will always prefer?

The problem is that we let the children eat only what they like and not what really fuels the body. . . without teaching them or explaining why? . . .

We as adults are primarily responsible for our children to provide the best food for them since they're little children. . .our duty to educate them about this without them feeling dominated or subjected, I emphasize that this is do be done with politeness. . .which in turn means more teaching with love and wisdom. . .

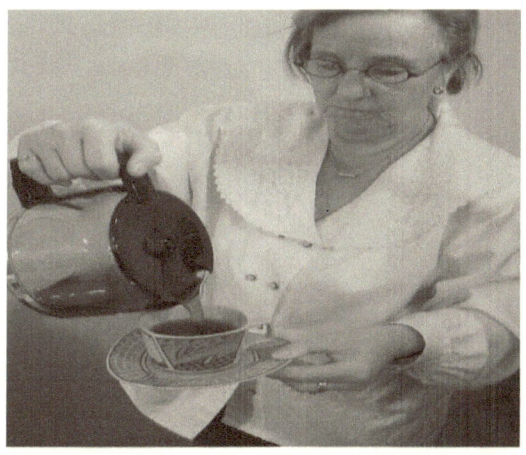

AS WE GET OLDER AND OUR PROBLEMS CONITUE, WE JUST KEEP EATING WHAT WE LIKE AND WE DO NOT EAT WHAT REALLY FEEDS US.

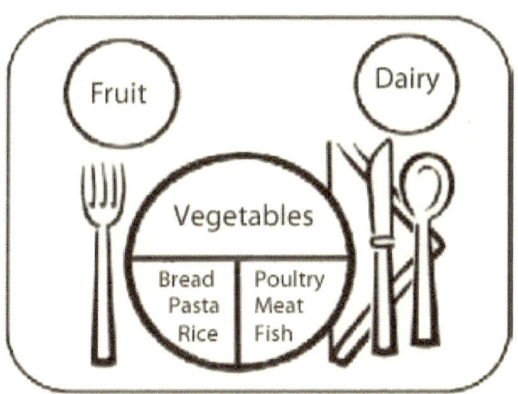

Who said a donut and coffee feeds you? "Sugar plus caffeine" and especially in the morning when the body needs all the nutrients of the day.

And like most everyone else who isn't eating well, we want to get all our nutrients through vitamin supplementation . . . just because they think that if there is no meat there is no food.

Good nutrition is based on that half the plate should be vegetables and the fruit serving should be eaten first and then the rest between proteins and grains. . .

MIXTURE OF GOOD FOOD

Another major problem is that we are accustomed to eating backwards, we begin;

Traditional:

We eat the main course of meats, breads, cheeses, etc. Then we eat we salads and fruit we save for dessert. ERROR! . . . if you eat fruits at the end it will produce heartburn, and this will feel like a jumble fermenting in the stomach, and we look to resolve it with an anti-acid. . . and incidentally we drink an abundant amount of water or soda with a lot of ice during and after eating which will only worsen situation. . .

The right way:

Don't drink water during or after meals. . . We can drink water 30 minutes before eating, and 45 or 60 minutes after eating, but are not during meals because the process of digestion is interrupted. The way to start is to eat fruits because fruits should be eaten on an empty stomach, because it's the intestine that digests fruits and absorbs all the nutrients, and most fruits are more than 50% water . . . then come the vegetables which is what nourishes the body most and gives combined energy with (lentils, beans, etc. energy. And finally the main course meats, protein, fish, cheeses and breads etc. should eat meat sparingly and only the size of the palm and once a week maximum and if you don't eat it even better. . .

WHEN TO DRINK WATER

Drinking water at the correct time maximizes its effectiveness on the human body

2 glasses of water after waking up helps activate the internal organs.
1 glass of water 30 minutes before a meal helps digestion.
1 glass of water before a bath helps lower blood pressure.
1 glass of water before going to bed avoids stroke or heart attack.

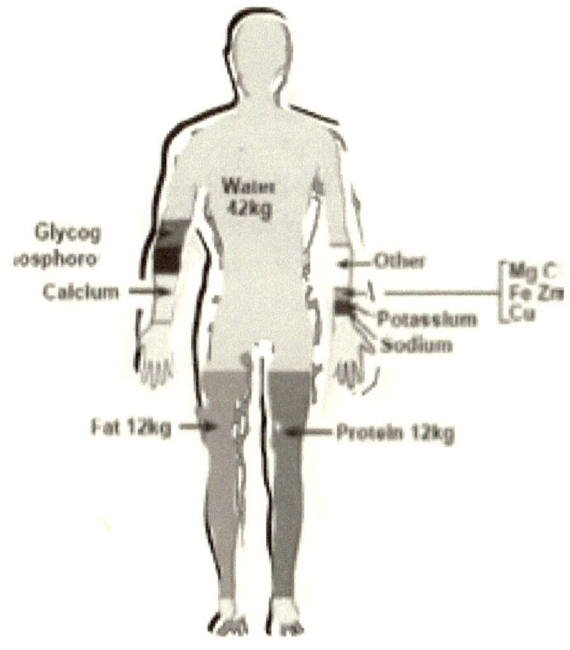

70% of the body is water

(I said NO Club soda or soda or artificial juices ...)

Turning now to the area of smokers

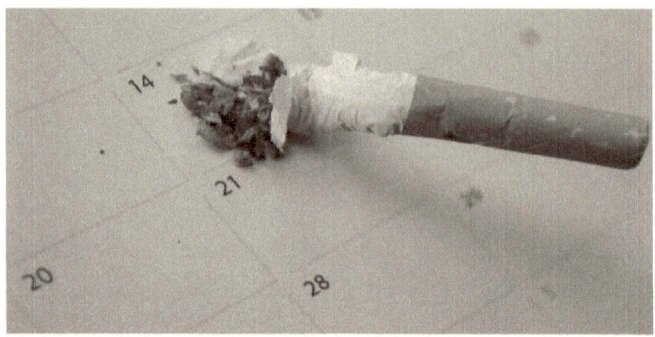

Take note on what is the smoking area? They are digging their own grave. . .

(Warnings)

It is now reported on the back of cigarette boxes that it is injurious to health, indicating that it especially causes lung cancer, also, causing heart problems, and too that pregnant women should not smoke as this would increase the risk that the child will be born with health problems or premature. . .

BUT WHO CARES?

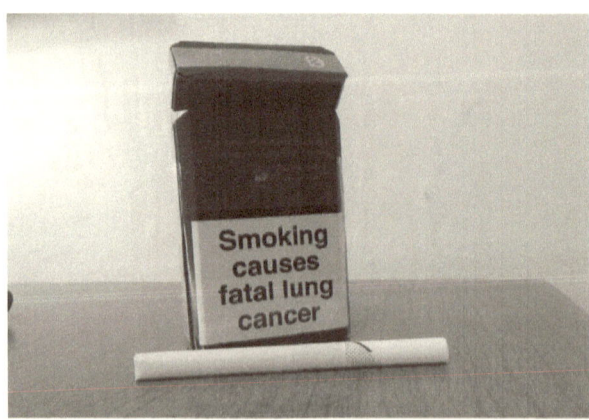

This is what it seems, at least to some people, they wait till they're on the brink of death to start making changes that should have been made much earlier. . . As always, we leave everything to the last hour including our own health.

Look at how a clean lung looks:

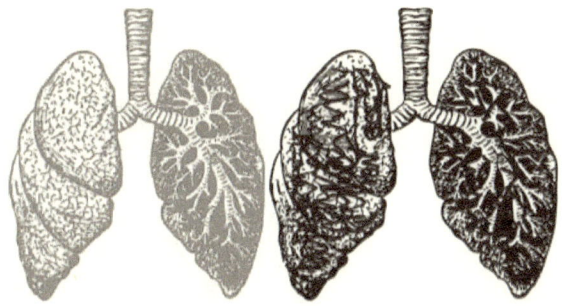

And notice the lungs of a person who lives with a smoker, what we call a second hand smoker (on the right), looks blotchy as if they smoked:

And then the lungs of a person who decided to be a smoker for life:

In 1960-1970 Marlboro man Wayne McLaren, at age 30, recorded this commercial (doesn't he look old for only being 30?) worn out by cigarettes.

Wayne McLaren died in 1992

He died at 52 yrs. old of lung cancer

Darrell Winfield Oklahoma1929- 1989 died of lung cancer at age 60.

Dick Hammer all died from lung cancer.

Eric Lawson, former 'Marlboro Man,' who appeared in ads for Marlboro cigarettes in the late 70s died Jan. 10, 2014 due to respiratory failure at the age of 72. Lawson, a former actor, also made his career appearing on many television shows...

These professional smoker models died of lung cancer, they were killed the same way by the same brand of cigarettes.

There was a commercial where it showed a cowboy smoking but what they did not realize at the time of shooting it, which there was much criticism, is that the model was a real smoker, so much so that his skin looked like a tobacco leaf and that kind of skin is a characteristic of those who smoke excessively. And the other, who was an expert in smoking, died shortly after of lung cancer, in fact both of them died to lung cancer. The first two. To which the advertising agency had to change the model to one that never in his life had smoked . . . and 1990 they came out with this new commercial, being careful about the details of past mistakes as seen in this photo.

Drugs

As drugs have also been the enemy of our health and have been uncontrollable for both those who consume it and for the government . . . with so many restrictions and yet it always sneaks into our community, but who cares about the drug addict's health . . .?

We know that drugs affect the brain directly, and destroy neurons which will never regenerate. There exists several types of drugs: antidepressants, stimulants, etc.

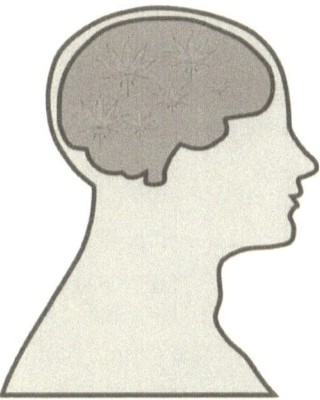

In the end they degenerate the human being to the point of losing their senses and losing many values.

Cerebral Nervous System connected to the body

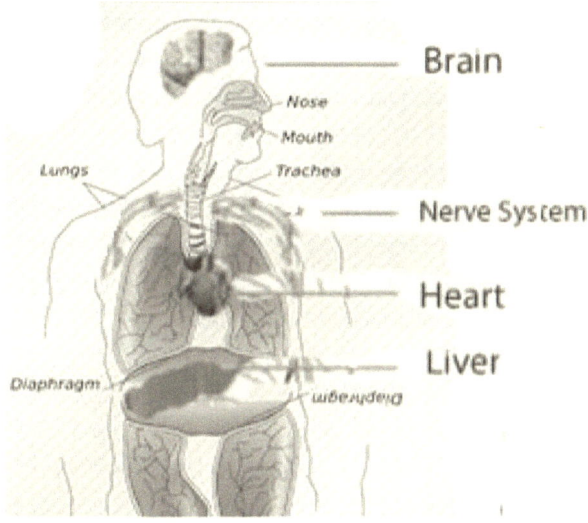

The nervous system is composed of a network of tissues and other various structures. It can be divided into four parts; the central nervous system, peripheral, autonomic and sympathetic or parasympathetic. The nervous system controls all organs of the body.

Drugs cause irreparable damage to the nervous system. They alter normal processes, cause destruction of the neurons and when a neuron is destroyed they cannot be replaced, since they are the only cells that do not reproduce. In the same way alcohol also damages many organs of the body.

Alcohol is a depressant substance of the nervous system. It affects the digestive, circulatory and respiratory systems, nutrition, skin, muscles and nervous system. In which the upper structures of the cerebral cortex are affected. And alcohol has more areas of destruction than prohibited drugs but this does not justify the use of either . . . especially the liver which cannot filter all the pollution and poisoning which goes to the brain. . . .

The point here is that it doesn't matter if it's minimal alcohol consumed, because its effects are equally negative.

And apart from the internal physical damage it does to your health, it also does psychological damage to your family and in most cases that you drink and drive, you go to jail.

Drinking and driving can cause accidents and drive where it always costs innocent victims. . . With regard to the laws of some countries like America there is severe punishment to the fullest of the law; drunk driving, regardless if it were just a few drinks, one is considered a potential murderer.

D.U.I. (Driving Under the Influence of alcohol or a narcotic substance) over 50% of accidents and deaths are caused by driving under the influence of alcohol. Upon receiving a DUI your license will revoked and you'll pay with jail time plus more costly fines.

Accidents caused by alcohol

About 50% of all accidents with two cars or more have been related to alcohol.

About 65% of individual accidents were also alcohol related.

About 36% percent of adult pedestrians killed in an accident was alcohol-related.

80% of all crashes caused between the hours of 8pm and 8am are related to alcohol.

36% of all pedestrian accidents were intoxicated by some form of drug.

About 20% of accidents of young people between 16 and 24 years old is caused by alcohol.

Moving on to another subject;

William Shakespeare said:

"SLEEP IS THE CHIEF NUTRIENT OF THE GREAT PARTY OF LIFE."(pg 157)

Everything has it's time... (a time to sleep...) (Ecclesiastes 3:1-9) The Bible "cease to sleep longer than is needful; retire to thy bed early, that ye may not be weary; arise early, that your bodies and your minds may be invigorated." (D&C 88:124)

"Six days shalt thou labour, and do all thy work" (but the seventh you should rest) (Exodus 20:9)

Do not run faster or labor more than you have strength (D&C 10:4)

All these are inspired writings and exist for a wise reason from our Creator, not obeying them doesn't bring human punishment, but punishment of your own health. . . Because sooner or later you be prematurely aged and unknown pains you shouldn't have so early in life. . .

Reasons to go to sleep early and wake early

9pm - 11pm: is the time in which the body removes unnecessary and toxic chemicals (detoxification) through the lymphatic system of the body. This part of the day should be used to find a relaxed state, listening to music, for example.

Usually at this time moms perform activities such as cleaning the kitchen, check to make sure everything is ready for the activities of the next day, etc. activities that create a state of lack of relaxation which generates a negative health effect.

11pm - 1:00 a.m. the body makes the detoxification process of the liver, and ideally should be done in a state of deep sleep.

During the early morning hours 1:00 a.m. to 3:00 a.m. is the process of the detoxification of the gallbladder. Ideally, this should also occur in a state of deep sleep.

Early morning 3:00 a.m. to 5:00 a.m. is the detoxification of the lungs. This is why sometimes this during these hours occurs a severe cough. When the detoxification process has reached the respiratory tract it is best not to take cough medicine being that it interferes with the process of removing toxins.

From 5:00 a.m. to 7:00 a.m. is the colon detox, it's the time to go the bathroom to empty the bowel. During the morning 7:00 a.m. to 9:00 a.m. is nutrient absorption in the small intestine, it's the perfect time for breakfast. If you are sick you should eat breakfast earlier, before 6:30 am. Breakfast before 7:30 am is beneficial for those who want to keep fit. Those who always skip breakfast should change their habit, at least eating between 9 and 10 a.m. is less harmful than skipping it all together.

Going to sleep late and waking up late will disrupt the process of removing unnecessary chemicals from your body. Also, you should keep in mind that from 12:00 to 4:00 am is the schedule in which the marrow of your bones produces blood, so try to sleep well and don't go to sleep late.

Fighting sleep while driving the car is also considered a D.U.I.

Give your body rest, it's the only machine that maintains you and so don't abuse it. . . Protect it them like the temple of God. . .

The pyramid of a healthy body

There are three parts that are balancing your entire health. . .

And these are: Macro-nutrients, Micro-nutrients and Water.

Pyramid of a Healthy Body

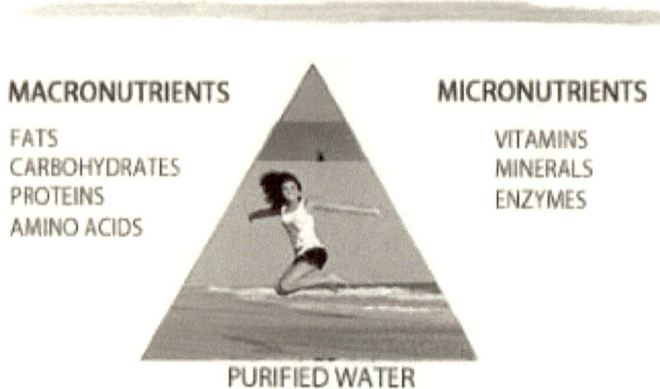

MACRONUTRIENTS

FATS
CARBOHYDRATES
PROTEINS
AMINO ACIDS

MICRONUTRIENTS

VITAMINS
MINERALS
ENZYMES

PURIFIED WATER

Macro-nutrients are composed of fats, carbohydrates, proteins and minerals.

Nutrition is defined as the science of food and its relationship to health. Food is made up of a broad distribution of nutrients that have very specific metabolic effects on the human body. Some of these nutrients are considered essential while others are considered non-essential. Essential nutrients are nutrients that cannot be synthesized by the human body and therefore must be derived from natural food sources. Essential nutrients include vitamins, minerals, amino acids, fatty acids and some carbohydrates as power source. Non-essential nutrients are nutrients that the body has the ability to synthesis from other compounds. Nutrients are generally divided into two categories, macro-nutrients and micro-nutrients. The macronutrients make up most of the diet of an individual, "Thereby providing energy and the essential nutrients required for growth, maintenance and activity" (2). Macronutrients are carbohydrates, proteins, fats, macro minerals and water. Carbohydrates, proteins and fats are interchangeable as sources of energy, fat producing 9 calories per gram and protein and carbohydrates each generate 4 calories per gram.

Micronutrients are vitamins and trace minerals.

Vitamins and trace minerals are labelled as micronutrients because the body only requires them in very small amounts. Vitamins are organic substances ingested with our food, and "act as catalysts, substances that help trigger other reactions in the body "Trace minerals are inorganic substances that once ingested play a role in a variety of metabolic processes and contribute to the synthesis of elements such as glycogen, protein and fat."

Each of these are important for the body and the correct functioning of each organ depends on balancing these foods which are needed in specific portions without abuse but must not be completely removed and the body needs each of these nutrients. . . (Unless your doctor prohibits them for reasons of health, illness or allergy)

HOW HUMAN CELLS DIE AND PREMATURE AGING

Free radicals are highly reactive molecules, and the result of these reactions generates a disruption in the cell membranes of our body. This disorder is lethal for the cell.

Moreover, free radicals also bind to various chemical substances in the body, among which is DNA, causing damage to the same.

Free radicals are molecules with an unpaired electron in its exterior orbit. In organic systems, there are two ways to produce free radicals: poor eating and environmental pollution.

Free radicals are highly reactive substances that cause a highly oxidizing peroxide reaction.

Free radicals: highly reactive chemical fragments that can cause irritation in the walls of arteries and initiate the arteriosclerosis process and lack of vitamin E.

Generally free radicals and oxidation are harmful.

Breathing in oxygen is essential for the cellular life of our body, but a consequence of the same produces some molecules, called free radicals which attack our bodies destroying it cellularly. . . As a result free radicals produce cellular oxidation.

Free radicals cause wrinkles in the skin, because of this vitamin E is helpful in cases of premature skin aging.

Free radicals are normal products of the metabolism of the body. However, in recent decades they have become the main cause of aging and degenerative damage, for two reasons: we have increased their presence (smoking, pollution and poor eating. . .)

It is now known that the process aging and the appearance of some diseases is due to the effect of "free radicals". That is, certain particles oxidizing our cells.

Free radicals also try to attack the appetite of neurons, but these are protected by the separation of two proteins (UCP2).

Anti-free radicals. Muscle, nerve, fat metabolism. . .

Nuts and their natural oils. Whole grain bread, fish, vegetables and vitamin H, E, omega 3 and anti-oxidants help counteract these free radicals and toxins. . .

Many of these free radicals produce diseases like cancer, diabetes, cardiovascular problems, etc. All these free radicals are triggered by smoking, alcohol, bad food, excess fat, environmental pollution, creating toxins in the body . . . and the only way to fight them is with antioxidants. And these antioxidants come from, especially, natural organic fruits; some prefer the antioxidant pills, ok let me tell you something: never ever will these synthetic antioxidant tablets compete against natural organic fruit. The chemical process to make pills, extracting antioxidant substances and elements, etc. doesn't even compare to natural fruit rich in antioxidants . . . and these are the true neutralizers of these free radicals that silently destroy your body . . .

Chlorophyll- chlorophyll molecules are necessary for the photosynthesis process, through which light is transformed into energy, but recently its antioxidant properties were discovered.

Chlorophyll produced by vegetables is liposoluble, while that which is chemically altered and is the base of the products sold in pharmacies and variety stores is water soluble. This means the second one has more difficulty being absorbed by the gastrointestinal system. Furthermore, the liposoluble chlorophyll amplifies its antioxidant properties because it contains beta carotene.

WHEN FAT ATTACKS

Newsweek did a story of a deep investigation of how fat attacks and protects the body from toxins,

- Health Crisis
- Toxicity
- Stress
- Poor Eating
- Obesity

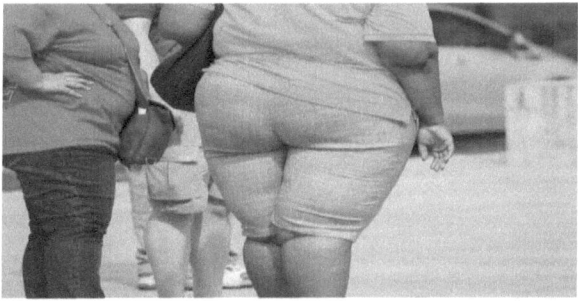

All these cause more fat to form in the body which attack the toxins produced by all these points . . . being a way of self-defense that the body itself created.

And this is one of the reasons why traditional diets do not work. . .

Traditional Diets vs. Internal Cleansing

Why don't traditional diets work? . . . People with excess body fat are full of impurities or toxins and they in turn try to lose weight

by taking miracle pills, fat burners, or liposuction and by removing
the excess fat quickly the body size is reduced and when reducing
the body and making it smaller, it will increase the impurities in
the body called toxins and in a smaller body the body sends a signal
automatically saying it needs more fat to protect itself from excess
impurities or toxins that destroy the body and that's where the
famous REBOUND comes from. . .

What would be the proper way to cut back naturally without
having a rebound?

The first thing to do is remove the impurities detoxifying our body
and if we do it naturally we need to go to a certified naturopathic
doctor, we could start by changing our poor eating, a colon cleanse,
rectal enema washes (do not use laxatives these damage intestinal
flora) using bags of warm water with a teaspoon of activated
charcoal, absinthe twigs and half a lemon squeezed in about two
liters of water. . . sauna baths (you can create your own sauna with
a small electric kitchen water pot with eucalyptus leaves and cover
yourself with a large plastic bag, sit on a chair and leaving just your
head exposed to be able to breathe properly. Keep the sides of the
plastic separated from the pot enough to not burn anything and
making sure to not cause any accident as shown in the illustration)
exercise regularly, cardio especially, fast for 24 hours once a month.

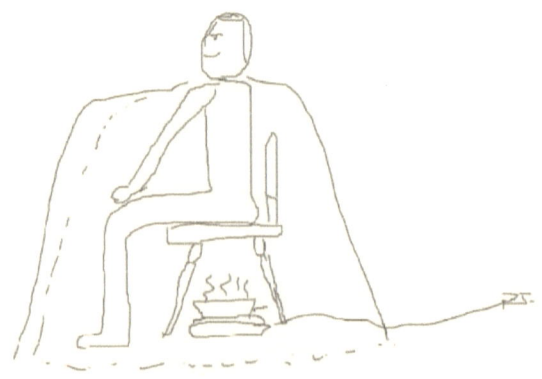

And perform ten days of the Daniel diet of only fruits, vegetables and water for 10 days, Drubinlife in the morning as breakfast and in the late afternoon as a substitute for dinner and lunch without meat or pork, no alcohol, no coffee, no cigarettes. . . This will prepare the way. . . (Remember to check with your doctor first before starting any diet) and if it is a naturopathic doctor they will indicate how to do a natural detox. There are also cleansings on a cellular level made by reputable companies; which have been very successful.

And by eliminating toxins your body will put off a signal of purity and automatically or naturally you'll be losing weight without regaining . . . and the muscle will be building to not let the skin hang. (if you add the correct cardio and muscle building weight).

59) A TIME BOMB

If you do not do something on time it has become a time bomb which can erupt at any time . . . for example if you stay sedentary (couch potato) alone watching TV eating all sorts of junk food you will be preparing for premature aging full of aches and pains causing problems not only for your body but also for others who have to look out for you.

60) TAKE CARE OF YOU BODY BEFORE IT'S TOO LATE

Maybe your body is sending you signals with various symptoms such as:

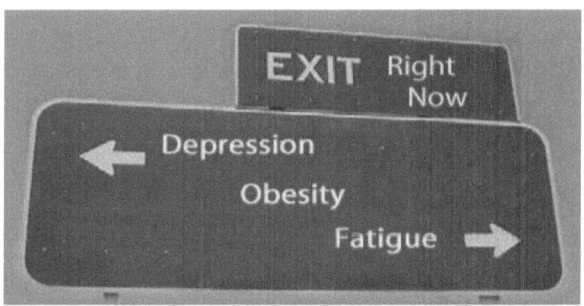

1. Frequent head aches
2. Heartburn
3. Constipation
4. Bad breath
5. Fatigue
6. Dizziness
7. Pain in bones bones
8. Arthritis
9. Diabetes
10. Tachycardia
11. Trouble Sleeping
12. Trouble breathing
13. Exhaustion with little effort
14. Obesity
15. Weakness
16. Spots on your skin
17. Impotence
18. Lack of appetite
19. Anxiety eating
20. Depression
21. Hair loss
22. Loss of sight at an early age
23. Bad Temper
24. Diarrhea

All these are signs just like when a you don't correctly maintain a vehicle nor change the oil or coolant to the radiator, or gas, there comes a time when lights begin to indicate the lack of something, and if we do not pay attention to these emergency lights, the vehicle and too, the body begins to fail. . . Sometimes many of us take better care of our car than our own body. We wash well the outside our body, but inside we put all the crap until it gives no more. . . Also, when we wait for the body to be thirsty it's too late because the body is at a point of dehydration and we forced it to wait for that signal. Our body must receive water daily without waiting for the signal of thirst, (ahead we'll give details on how and when to drink water) and most of these signs are late because when the oil light lights up it's because it's on the last drops of oil and could rupture the gears that drive the motor and could burn it up which then it would be too late and would never function again . . . the same with the radiator, when the temperature light turns on it's because it's about to overheat and you must stop the vehicle immediately or the machine will burn. . .

And someday when life takes its toll, it will be too late . . . do something for your life and health, this is the right time don't wait for these signals to arrive before doing something.

Hurry and make a radical change starting today with drubinlife, here in this book, pleading for you to take control of your life and to not wait to have a doctor tell you; you can no longer smoke, and you cannot eat meat, you cannot eat sweets, you cannot drink any more alcohol, etc. . . .

Why wait for it to happen this way? . . . if we don't care for this temple, no one else will do it for you, we are not machines that can be easily fixed and continue as usual. . . although today there are many organ transplants I'm sure if you have not already come to that, that you don't want another operation because of the self-abuse of your body.

61) STAY OBEDIANT IN FOLLOWING THE WORD OF WISDOM

The old food pyramid showed us how to balance food. . . indicating that in the tip to take small portions;

Old Pyramid

OLD FOOD PYRAMID

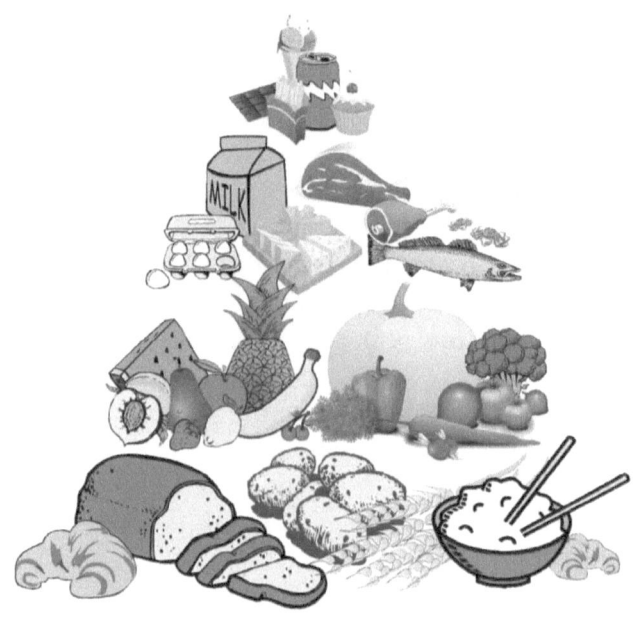

1. Fats, oils and sweets eaten in moderation. . .
2. Milk yogurt and cheese 2-3 servings // Meat, poultry, fish, dry beans, eggs and nuts 2-3 servings. . .
3. Vegetables 3-5 servings // Fruit 2-4 servings. . .
4. Bread, cereal, rice and pasta 6-11 servings. . .

This food pyramid has been around for many years and recently was changed to one that is closer to current reality. . .

NEW FOOD PYRAMID

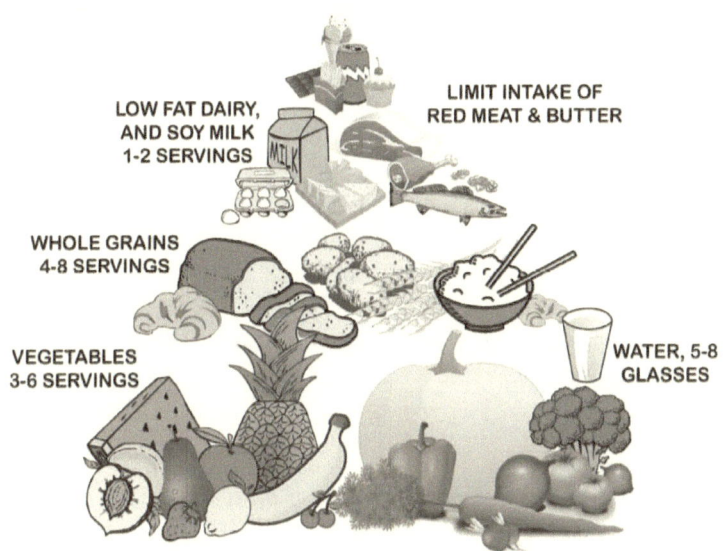

LOW FAT DAIRY, AND SOY MILK 1-2 SERVINGS

LIMIT INTAKE OF RED MEAT & BUTTER

WHOLE GRAINS 4-8 SERVINGS

VEGETABLES 3-6 SERVINGS

WATER, 5-8 GLASSES

DAILY EXERCISE AND WEIGHT CONTROL

Starting at the top;

1. Red meat goes to the top where you should be eating less and with moderation, in other words, the revelation of more than 150 years ago given to Joseph Smith is fulfilled when God told him;
2. MEAT HAVE I ORDAINED FOR THE USE OF MAN. . . NEVERTHELESS GTHEY ARE TO BE USED SPARINGLY; AND IT IS PLEASING UNTO ME THAT THEY SHOULD NOT BE USED. . . ONLY IN TIME OF WINTER OR OF COLD OR FAMINE . . . February 1833. . .
3. Also, in that area, it speaks of butter and all types of fried food. . .

4. Low-fat milk or soy milk and talks about multivitamins . . . perhaps because nowadays people have to use vitamin supplements for lack of eating good food.
5. Water 5-8 cups daily . . . /// Eggs, fish, poultry from one 1-2 portions. . .
6. Oats, grains, nuts, seeds 1-2 servings. . .
7. Whole wheat bread, corn and its derivatives 2-6 servings. . .
8. Olive oil, avocado and its derivatives 2-4. . .
9. Plants of 4-8 servings . . . fruit 2 to 4 servings (Drubinlife)
10. Add in exercise and weight control. . .

You may have noticed that bread is reduced one level and says it must be whole grain bread . . . because of its fiber, it's more food and reduces sugars. . .

Vegetables and fruits also moved to the most important level and larger portions . . . no coffee, no alcohol, no smoking, no drugs, or carbonated soft drinks, or the sweeteners appear in this pyramid. . .

All this helps further your health and confirms that the health revelations of 1833. . . are true. . .

1 Corinthians 3:16-17 Know ye not that ye are the temple of God, and *that* the Spirit of God dwelleth in you? If any man defile the temple of God, him shall God destroy; for the temple of God is holy, which *temple* ye are.

The word of wisdom is a valuable temporal law and also a spiritual law, it strengthens our temple so that the Holy Spirit dwells in us. . . Gospel Principles Book

DRINK THE DRUBINLIFE SMOOTHIE DAILY

Nothing and I mean NOTHING, It's that NOTHING can replace the fiber-rich juice, fresh and nutritious enzymes that is received from a smoothie with plant vegetables and fruits directly from your blender. . . (Drubinlife)

THAT YOUR FOOD BE YOUR MEDICINE AND YOUR MEDICINE BE YOUR FOOD...

Hippocrates; the Father of Medicine (500 B.C.)

HERE'S THE SOLUTION TO ALL DISEASE, THE FAMOUS "DRUBINLIFE"

INGREDIENTS IN DRUBINLIFE:

CELERY,	GREEN APPLE,
GREEN BEENS,	GREEN GRAPES,
SPINACH,	KIWI,
WATERCRESS,	MANGO,
CARROTS,	STRAWBERRY,
LETTUCE,	BANANA,
CACTUS W/O NEEDLES	PEAR,
AVOCADO,	RABANO,
CUCUMBER,	ASPARAGUS,
BROCCOLI.	

Preparation; MIX ALL WITH APPLE JUICE INCLUDING THE SKINS AND SEEDS (except apple seeds, avocado and mango. . .) (REMEMBER TO CONSULT WITH YOUR DOCTOR)

Each of these fruits and vegetables contain all the properties your body needs in a day . . . this will be your breakfast from now on if you want to live longer and healthier. . . Here I emphasize the famous natural vegetable recipe V10G- 10 combined vegetables. . .

INGREDIENTS V10G

CELERY	BEET
SPINACH	WATERCRESS
CARROTS	LETTUCE
RABANO	TOMATO
PURPLE CABBAGE	PARSLEY

Preparation; FOR THIS YOU'LL NEED A JUICER, MIX ALL WITH TOMATO JUICE AND A TOUCH OF LEMON, SALT AND BLACK PEPPER TO TASTE

(REMEMBER TO CHECK WITH YOUR DOCTOR to make sure you can take it even though most of these are not contrdictive.) I use this V10G especially for dinner. . . now for mid-morning: flaxseed stew.

FLAXSEED STEW INGREDIENTS:

Almonds	Flaxseed
Bran (whole grain wheat)	Wheat germ
Oats	Plums
Honey	Water
Peanut Butter	

Preparation: SOAK ALL THESE INGREDIENTS IN WATER THE NIGHT BEFORE EATING IT. MIX WITH BLENDER AND DRINK IT ALL NATURAL... (REMEMBER TO CHECK WITH YOUR DOCTOR)

25 Years of Health

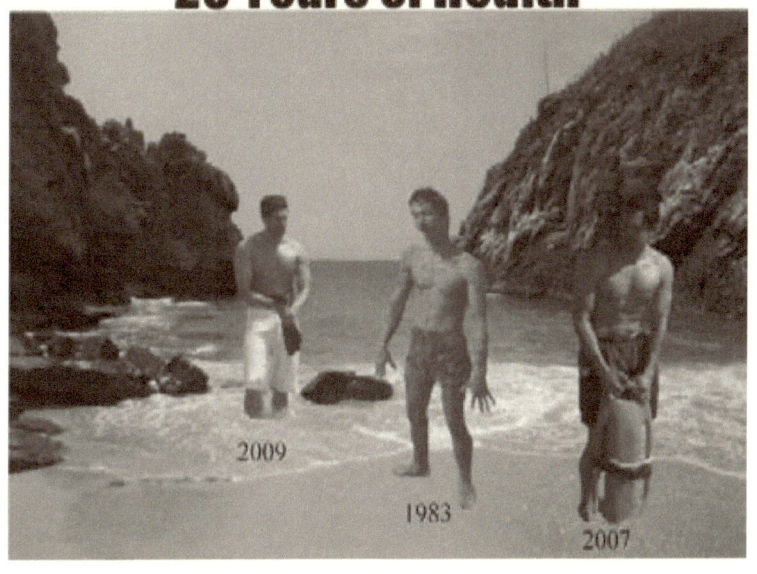

2009

1983

2007

GREEN, OH HOW I LOVE GREENS... THE POWER OF GREENS

POWERFUL FRUITS

A sliced carrot looks like the human eye. The pupil, iris and radiating lines look just like the human eye . . . and YES, science now shows that carrots greatly enhance blood flow to the eyes and their function.

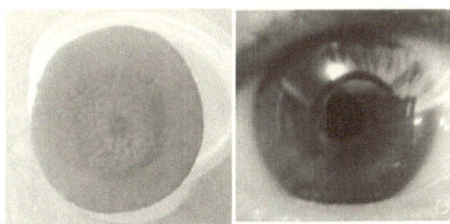

A tomato has four chambers and is red. The heart is red and has four chambers. Research shows that tomatoes are a pure food good for the heart and blood.

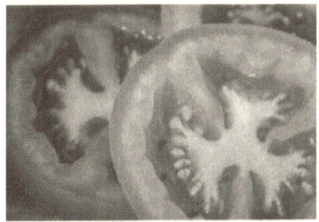

Grapes hang in a cluster that has the shape of the heart. Each grape looks like a blood cell and research today shows that grapes are a vitalizing food for the heart and blood.

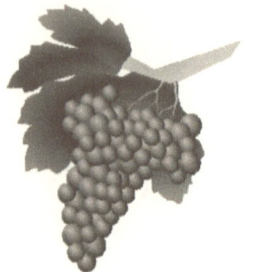
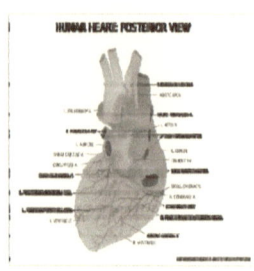

A Walnut looks like a little brain, a left and right hemisphere, upper and lower brains. Even the wrinkles or folds are located in the same place as the cerebral cortex. We know that walnuts help develop more than 3 dozen neuro-transmitters for brain function.

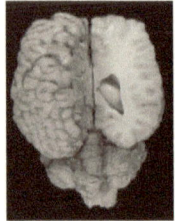
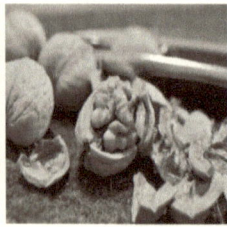
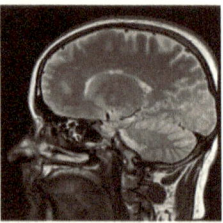

Beans actually heal and help maintain kidney function and yes, they look exactly like human kidneys.

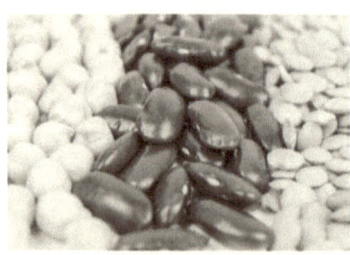
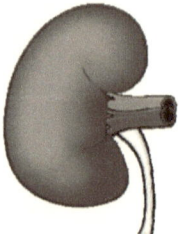

Celery, rhubarb, Bok Choy and others resemble bones. These foods are aimed specifically at strengthening bones. Bones are 23% sodium and these foods are 23% sodium. If you do not have enough sodium in your diet the body pulls it from the bones, making them weak. These foods replenish the skeletal needs of the body.

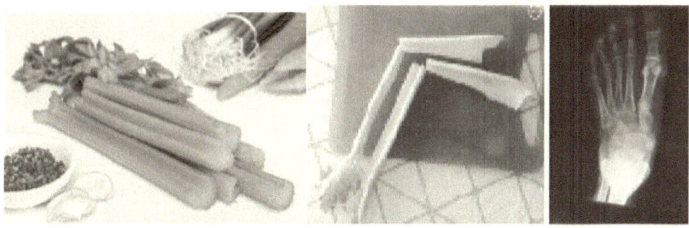

Eggplant, Avocados and Pears target the health and operation of the uterus and cervix – and they resemble these organs. Today's research shows that when a woman eats one avocado a week, it balances hormones, sheds the unwanted baby weight and prevents cervical cancers. And how profound is this? . . . It takes exactly nine months to grow an avocado from blossom to ripened fruit. There are more than 14,000 photoliticosen chemical constituents in each of these foods (modern science has only studied and named 141 of them).

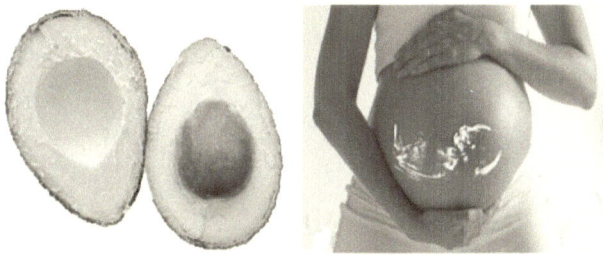

Figs are full of seeds and hang in pairs as they grow. Figs increase the mobility of sperm and increase sperm count, as well, to help reduce male infertility.

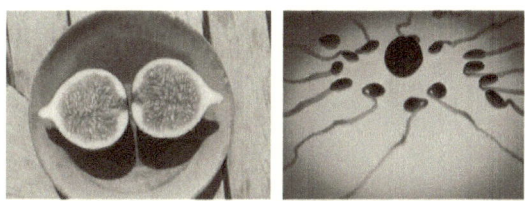

Sweet Potatoes look like the pancreas and actually balance the diabetic glycemic index.

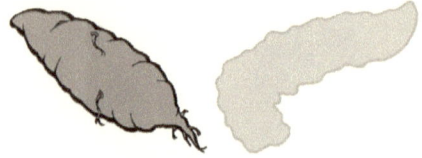

Olives assist the health and function of the ovaries.

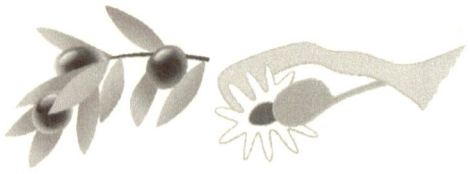

Grapefruits, Oranges and other citrus fruits look just like women breast glands and actually assist the health of the breasts and lymphatic movement to and from the breasts.

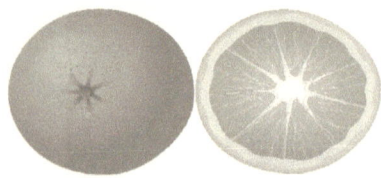

Onions look like body cells. Today research shows that onions help clear waste materials of body cells. They even produce tears which wash the epithelial layers of the eyes.

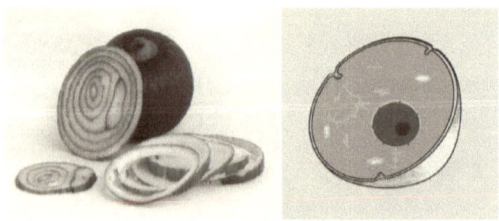

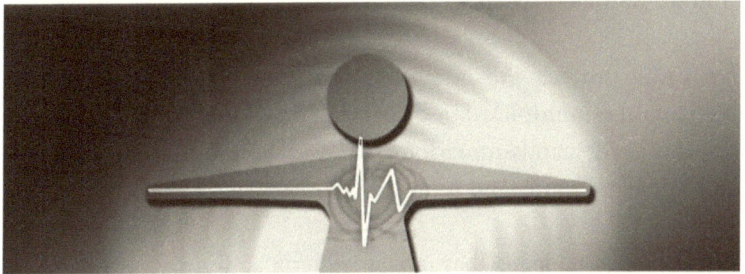

The Alkaline Miracle

Our bodies house a large amount of bacteria and fungi that live, grow and survive in harmony when we are eating and living healthy. But they can become very harmful when the environment where they live is altered.

This alteration of the environment is encouraged by diets high in sugar or carbohydrates also from contaminated water and air, or even the destruction of our intestinal flora because of the use of antibiotics or other medications.

Bacteria and fungi feed on the same substances as our brain.

When we eat too much food rich in glucose, we are also fueling excess bacteria and fungi which will grow and multiply disproportionately.

The consumption of these substances in excess which disproportionately overpopulate us causes the brain to not receive enough food, and since the brain is king it immediately issues orders demanding its share.

That is when we feel the urge to run and eat something sweet, carbohydrates (turns into glucose), or alcohol.

And so the vicious circle begins:

By eating more, the provisions of sugar grow, and thereby increases the multiplication of bacteria and fungi, and the growing population demands more food and we feel the need to eat more, and more and more, and more.....

But it just so happens that just as bacteria and fungi get their food from our blood, they also dump their waste in it too, the toxins become increasingly acidic and they eventually become a "poison" to the tissues.

In order to process the toxins, the liver converts them to alcohol (acid) and with that excess of alcohol in our body, we produce a feeling of being drunk ... dizzy, disoriented, and mentally confused.

Excessive accumulation of bacteria and fungi reduce the provision of potassium and magnesium in the body with consequent reduction in cellular energy that causes excessive fatigue, reduced strength and clarity of thought, removes enthusiasm, ambition, and stamina; and causes the release of free radicals which contribute to the aging process.

Other symptoms of accumulation of bacteria and fungi are panic attacks, anxiety, depression, irritability, headaches, joint pain, swelling in respiratory passages, sinusitis, glandular stress and menstrual problems.

Many scientific studies have coincided in that bacteria and fungi cause diseases when allowed to develop in unhealthy soil (acid).

Through various scientific studies, analyzing living blood cells, bacterial forms have been observed that live in our body (some even work to help the body) which depending on the environment in which they developed, sometimes grew and lengthened becoming pathogenic. In some cases, mutating from "bacteria" to "mushroom".

Few know it but...

Acidity in the pH of the tissues of our body is usually the hallmark of cancer and other imbalances of our health such as: cardiovascular diseases, cerebrovascular problems, pathologies of kidneys, inflammatory disorders and lung diseases.

Researcher Sang Whang, with 50 years of experience in the study of acid-alkaline balance, argues that: It is the excess of acid in our body that cultivates cancer, and makes the following assumptions:

1) Healthy cells are alkaline.
2) An acidic environment contains less oxygen than an alkaline environment.
3) Healthy cells die in an acidic environment, while cancer cells die in an ALKALINE environment.

He suggests that every cancer treatment should start by changing the acidic environment to an alkaline environment.

Dr. Robert O. Young, currently the most recognized microbiologist worldwide coincides with many scientists that: "Disease is the expression of excess acids in the human body."

Robert O. Young is a Doctor of Medicine, Microbiology and Nutrition.

For 30 years he has been performing analysis of living and dried blood, and his cancer research has been validated by a British scientific study. Daily, he caters to 14 patients in his Center "pH Miracle" located near San Diego, CA.

His protocol "Alkaline Lifestyle" has a 100% effectiveness in those who have applied and have managed to reverse a number of metabolic diseases.

Dr. Young, creator of the concept "New Biology", is the author of recognized bestsellers: "The pH Miracle", "Sick and Tired", "The pH Miracle for Diabetes", "The pH Miracle for Weight Loss" and "The pH Miracle for cancer".

As with more and more scientists, Dr. Robert O. Young argues that:

"Our organism manufactures and utilizes baking soda as a natural system to maintain the alkaline design to prevent tissue degeneration." (We recall the characteristic flavor of baking soda often times prior to vomiting)

"The hyper-alkalization of body tissues with sodium bicarbonate is the most safe, effective and natural way to stop any cancerous condition and many diseases and inflammatory processes and more"

For years Dr. Tullio Simmoncini, Italian oncologist, has been treating cancer and destroying tumors by using baking soda.

Dr. Simmoncini manifests; "Baking Soda is a sure remedy, extremely cheap and undeniably effective when it comes to cancerous tissues."

Most of us start our lives as healthy beings. As we age, and largely because of our unhealthy life styles, bacteria and fungi are constantly accumulating in our bodies, turning a healthy balance into vicious cycle, getting increasingly serious.

Bacteria and fungi poison, stress and weaken our immune system, and it is proven that most immunological diseases and infectious conditions are caused or worsened by the presence of bacteria and fungi.

Dr. Robert Young manifests:

"For years I have observed the impact of what we eat on the delicate pH balance of our blood. And through my investigations have shown that the combination of 4 wonderful bicarbonate salts (sodium, magnesium, potassium and calcium) occur naturally in all fluids of a healthy body, with the purpose to maintain the natural alkaline-acid balance and acting as anti-oxidants which retard the aging process. An adequate supply of these four bicarbonate salts is the best protection against aging and every disease, including cancer in addition to improving athletic performance and to improve overall health, and also to improve the state of mood and energy.

"During the recent Olympic Games in Beijing, several major athletes improved their performance and even managed to break some records, ingesting 1 tablespoon of baking soda"

To slow aging and restore health it's necessary to reverse the damage of acid in the cells by an alkalizing diet.

It's time to make the necessary changes in our way of life for our body comes back to a state of balance and harmony.

Maintain a Diet with a Majority % of Alkaline Foods

Most Alkaline	Medium Alkaline	Low Alkaline	Foods	Low Acid	Medium Acid	Most Acid
broccoli; cucumber; cilantro; oriental greens; garlic; onions; kale; spinach; parsley; sea vegetables; greens + "green drink"	bell pepper; cauliflower; parsnip; endive; ginger root; sweet potato; cabbage; celery; carrots; asparagus	Brussel sprouts; beets; tops & roots; tomatoes & tomatoe juice; fresh peas; dark lettuce; all mushrooms; fresh potato w/skin; pumkin; squash; tempeh	Vegetables, Beans, Legumes only use non-GMO foods	corn; lentils; peanuts w/skin; organic peanut butter; soy protein powder; beans: kidney, lima navy, pinto, white, black; peas: green; split & chick; tofu (extra firm); edamame	salted peanut butter	processed soybeans; salted & sweetened peanut butter
cantaloupe; honeydew; raisins; nectarine; raspberry; watermelon; fresh black cherries; black olives in oil	apple; avocado; pink grapefruit; lemons; limes; mangoes; pear; peach	fresh pineapple; apricot; grapes; blueberry; strawberry; blackberry; papaya	Fruits	dried fruit; natural figs; dates; prunes; banana; unsweetened canned fruit; natural fruit juice; unsweetened jams; unsweetened preserves	olives; pickles; sweetened fruit juice; sweetened canned fruit; sweetened jams; sweetened preserves	cranberry; dried fruit; sulfured
Celtic sea salt; RealSalt (Great Salt Lake); miso & natto; cayenne; ashwagandha; gotu kola; ginkgo biloba; baking soda (sodium bicarbonate)	cinnamon; ginger; dill; mint; peppermint; turmeric; rhodiola; basil; oregano; licorice root; Siberian ginseng	most herbs; curry; mustard powder; kola nut; tamari; milk thistle; maca; astragalus; suma; echinacea	Seasonings Herbs, Spices	tahini; carob; cocoa; regular table salt	vanilla; nutmeg; mayonnaise; ketchup	black pepper; MSG; soya sauce; brewer's & nutritional yeast
electon-rich alkaline water; plasma activated water (PAW)	Teas: green, matcha green, ginger; rooibos; chamomile; water; ozonated water; ionized water	dry red wine; unsweetened almond milk; distilled water; beer (draft) or dark stout; black coffee (organic)	Beverages	unsweetened soy milk; unsweetened rice milk; black tea; black coffee; decaf coffee	coffee (milk & sugar)	alcoholic drinks; soft drinks
bee pollen; soy lecithin granules; dairy-free probiotic cultures	aloe vera juice	whole oats; quinoa; wild rice; millet & spelt; hemp protein powder	Grains Cereals, Other	brown & basmati rice; wheat & buckwheat; kasha; amaranth; whole wheat & corn pasta; whole grain bread	plain rice protein powder; rolled oats & oat bran; rye; white bread; white pasta; white rice	barley; pastries; cakes; tarts; cookies
pumpkin seeds; almonds w/skin; plain almond butter w/skin; all sprouts; wheat grass; alfalfa grass; barley grass	extra virgin olive oil; borage oil & primrose oil; chestnuts; nuts: Brazil & macadamia; light & dark flaxseeds; black currant oil	hazelnuts; flaxseed & sea buckthorn oils; hemp seeds & oil; sesame seeds & oil; sunflower seeds & oil; fresh coconut & oil	Nuts & Seeds, Grasses & Sprouts, Oils	popcorn; canola oil; grape seed oil; green soybeans; pine nuts; safflower oil	cashews; pecans; walnuts	pistachios; trans fatty acids; acrylamides
	wild; ultra-pure omega3 fish oil CLA (conjugated linoleic acid)	cod liver oil	Meats Fish & Fowl	fish; turkey; venison; wild duck; seafood	chicken; lamb; pork; veal	beef; lobster
human breast milk	dairy probiotic cultures; whey protein isolate powder	soft goat cheese; fresh goat milk	Dairy, Eggs	cow's milk; cream; yogurt; butter; buttermilk; white of chicken eggs	soy cheese & soft cheese; ice cream; whole chicken eggs	processed cheese; hard cheese; yolk of chicken eggs
	(unsulfured) blackstrap molasses	stevia; brown rice syrup; pure maple syrup; unpasteurized honey	Sweeteners	commercial honey	corn syrup & fructose; high-fructose corn syrup; sugar	artificial sweeteners
	apple cider vinegar		Vinegar	rice vinegar	balsamic vinegar	white vinegar

Drink at least one liter of water per day to which you have added a tablespoon of baking soda.

This will help flush out your system and liberate it from the accumulated acidity.

To revert cases of pneumonia, asthma, sinusitis, make nebulized water with two drops of liquid baking soda, 2 or 3 times a day.

To prevent bacterial accumulation in the mouth, swish a blend of a teaspoon of baking soda in a glass of water.

To remove residual chemicals in your hair, add a teaspoon of baking soda to your shampoo bottle.

According to Dr. Robert O. Young: "if we keep our body with an alkaline pH between 7.3 and 7.4 we will remain disease free."

Take your baking soda every day...

<u>THIS IS TRUE PREVENTION</u>

http://www.phmiracleliving.com/pHourSalts.htm

SYMPTOMS WHICH APPEAR WITH AGE AND HOW TO TREAT THEM...

The latter is the most difficult to achieve. . .

Symptoms caused by need of some foods;

Look how interesting . . . after a certain age, we have almost all of these symptoms, caused by a lack of food mentioned below.

1. **DIFFICULTLY LOSING WEIGHT.**

WHAT'S LACKING: Essential fatty acids and vitamin A. WHERE TO GET THEM: flaxseed, carrots and salmon – plus specific supplements.

2. **FLUID RETENTION**

WHAT'S LACKING: Indeed, it's an imbalance between potassium, phosphorus and sodium. WHERE TO GET THEM: coconut water, olive, peach, plum, fig, almond, nuts, spinach, cilantro and supplements.

3. <u>NEED FOR SWEETS</u>

WHAT'S MISSING: Chromium

WHERE TO GET IT: Whole grains, walnuts, rye, banana, spinach, carrot, and supplements.

4. <u>CRAMP, HEADACHE</u>

WHAT'S MISSING: Potassium and magnesium.

WHERE TO GET THEM: banana, barley, corn, peaches, acerola, orange, tomato and water.

5. <u>INTESTINAL IRRITATION, GAS, ABDOMINAL SWELLING</u>

WHAT'S MISSING: Live bacilli

WHERE TO GET IT: curd, yogurt, Yakult and the like.

6. <u>BAD MEMORY</u>

WHAT'S MISSING: Acetylcholine, inositol

WHERE TO GET THEM: Soy lecithin, egg yolk and supplements.

7. <u>HYPOTHYROIDISM</u> (CAUSES WEIGHT GAIN WITHOUT AN APPARENT CAUSE)

WHAT'S MISSING: iodine

WHERE TO GET: seaweed, carrot oil, pear, pineapple, salt water fish with scales and sea salt.

8. <u>BRITTLE HAIR AND FRAGILE NAILS</u>

WHAT'S MISSING: collagen.

WHERE TO GET: fish, eggs, lean meat, gelatin and supplements.

9. <u>THINNESS, MALAISE, DISCOMFORT</u>

WHAT'S MISSING: Vitamins A, C, and E and iron.

WHERE TO GET THEM: vegetables, fruits, lean meats and supplements.

10. <u>LOW MORALE, APATHY, SADNESS, DISATISFACTION</u>

WHAT'S MISSING: money. . .

WHERE TO GET IT: If you know where to find it, please let me know, don't be selfish; look at all the information I have given you so that you're healthy . . . haha take care of your health☺

PROPERTIES OF NUTRITIONAL YEAST

For many years yeast has been part of man's diet. In some cultures, it was used to complement a variety of foods and beverages, due to its ability to improve the nutritional profile of the same. Brewer's yeast is a product which is obtained during the manufacturing of the beverage but doesn't contain alcohol. Basically, it is a ferment from the decomposition of barley and isn't anything but dry cells and a crushed up fungus known as Saccharomyces cerevisiae, which has no repercussion on the health of people but rather the opposite. Also, the yeast can be grown in laboratories for specific use as a nutritional supplement. However, it is likely that this product does not have the same nutritional value as the yeast obtained by the fermentation of barley during the preparation of this drink.

Because the process of obtaining brewer's yeast, it has a very bitter taste, which is unpleasant for many consumers, which is subjected to a "washing" process that seeks to eliminate this flavor. Thus, two types of yeast are commercially known: Bitter and debittered. Basically the amount of nutrients in these two types of food are the same and only very detailed studies can show that bitter yeast contains only a slightly higher nutrient value.

It is a supplement rich in proteins and B vitamins, along with a variety of minerals. It is ideal to supplement deficient diets, and is easy to digest and absorb in our body. The protein content of the yeast is the most important nutritional element, thus it makes up approximately 40% of its composition. Brewer's yeast has twice the amount of proteins as oilseed proteins found in such foods as almonds, walnuts and hazelnuts, and is matched only by eggs and milk. It also contains all amino acids considered essential by the World Health Organization. It should be noted the high content of two amino acids: lysine, which supports normal growth and bone development in children and adults, and tryptophan, which is very helpful for sleep.

Consuming 20-30 grams of yeast provides an adult weighing 150 lbs. between 15 and 17% of the recommended daily intake of protein, this implies that the yeast protein supplement is quite useful in vegetarian diets or simply low calorie diets deficient in this nutriment.

Brewer's yeast is the largest natural source of folic acid and is rich in other B vitamins such as B1, B2, niacin (B3), pantothenic acid (B5), B6 and biotin (B8), all these are essential for the normal development of cell functions during growth and reproduction, but are also important for protective and regenerative action of our nervous system.

Recent studies have shown that supplementation with dry yeast, fully or partially overcomes deficiencies of iron, copper, zinc, chromium, selenium, and molybdenum that certain diets sometimes have. As if that were not enough, its content in phosphorus, calcium, sulfur, manganese and silicon, is also important. Nutritionists recommend its consumption to those suffering from anemia, as well as growing children and adolescents being that it favors the formation of distinct hormones. Similarly, athletes found in brewer's yeast an ally to improve performance, because coupled with its high protein, it facilitates oxygenation of muscle tissue.

I cannot fail to mention that one of the properties most important in the yeast is that its composition is a biologically active form of chromium known as glucose tolerance factor (GTF) which has been shown to improve glucose tolerance and increase the effectiveness of the insulin hormone, revealing its benefits in the treatment of people who have diabetes mellitus. Likewise, there is reliable scientific information which states that after the consumption of brewer's yeast supplementation, it has been observed a decrease in circulating cholesterol in the blood.

In addition to the nutritional content as described, brewer's yeast has a certain tonic and cleanser effect. It fights the feelings of tiredness and has been credited with the ability to improve the state of skin, nails and hair. Finally, yeast helps regulate bowel function by participating in the renewal of bacterial flora and contains active substances which aid in maintaining the body's defenses, improving the immune system.

Because of all these characteristics, yeast is a comprehensive supplement from the nutritional point of view, ideal to supplement the diet of the people mentioned above, plus elderly people with inadequate food and generally anyone looking to improve the quality of their diet. Particularly, I recommend brewer's yeast either in powder, capsules or tablets, because they use pharmaceutical grade raw materials and is a product produced under strict quality standards, ensuring all the benefits of this food.

It also helps the growth and resilience of the hair loss. In the morning mix it with natural tamarind juice.

HOW TO CARE FOR YOUR SKIN

Performing an appropriate cosmetic treatment is the mainstay in anti-aging from age 30 and even more in your 50's. However, there is a number of extra care remedies specialists recommend to reduce the signs of aging and lack of estrogens:

Sunscreen: Use sunscreen UVA and UVB throughout the year, degree of protection varies according to the age and quality of sunshine that you are exposed to.

Hydration: Drink between 1.5 and 2 liters of water per day.

Exfoliation: in addition to daily cleansing, do cosmetic peels to promote the elimination of dead cells and to cleanse pores. The skin stays brighter, elastic and homogeneous.

Healthy Living: Keep a balanced diet rich in vitamins and fiber, regular physical activity, avoid alcohol and caffeine, and avoid smoking altogether.

HOW TO READ FOOD NUTRITIONAL LABELS

I know, you're probably thinking, "who has time to read food labels while you're shopping at the supermarket?"

It may take a minute the first time you attempt to read or even glance at the label, but once you identify things you usually buy, the next time will be a breeze. You will also be relieved knowing that you are buying only the best foods and drinks for you and your family.

LEARN TODAY, BENEFIT FOR A LIFETIME

Invest in the health of your family. Plan to go to the supermarket for two hours, only once, paying close attention to food labels. These two hours will save you money and time besides protecting the health of your family.

We suggest you:

Go without the kids. The least amount of distraction the better.

Eat before you go. Hunger can be a great distraction. Invite someone like your sister or friend who is interested in improving their health because learning together is more fun.

Bring paper and pen to take note of healthy products to try out or to just take notes.

READING FOOD LABELS

There are 7 main elements that should be reviewed on a food label. This is what you should know about each one of them:

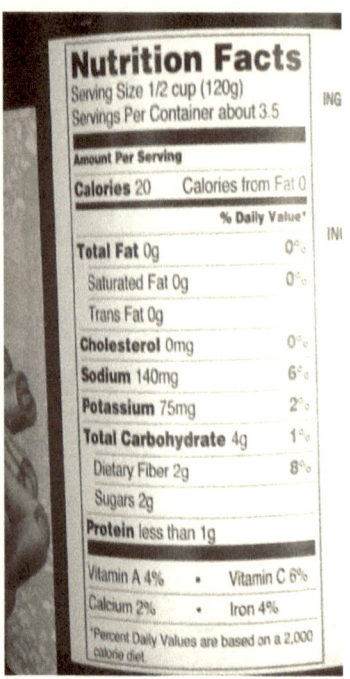

PORTION SIZE

Start by checking the serving size. The label describes the nutritional value of the proportion size, not the whole package. For example, if the label on a packet of pasta says the ration is a cup and you usually eat two cups of pasta you have to double the nutritional information.

CALORIES

The average person should consume about 2000 calories a day. If you're not active you should consume less calories. It sounds like it is a lot, but a McDonald's Big Mac meal (with the Big Mac, fries and a medium coke) contains 1130 calories. This is more than half the calories you should consume in a day. Remember that calories on the label only correspond to the portion size and not the whole package. You must divide up calories consumed throughout the day.

TOTAL FAT (including saturated and trans fats)

Total fat indicates the amount of fat in a serving of the product being reviewed. This includes healthy fats the body needs (monounsaturated and polyunsaturated) and fats that are not healthy, whose consumption should be limited (saturated fat and trans fats.) Remember to limit the intake of saturated fats and avoid all Trans fats.

SODIUM AND CHOLESTEROL

Limit the consumption of cholesterol and sodium. The American Heart Association describes cholesterol as a substance that is soft and waxy found in torrent blood lipids (fats) and in all cells of the body. It is an important part of a healthy body because it's used to form cell membranes, some hormones and is needed for other functions. However, a high level of blood cholesterol is a major risk factor for coronary heart disease, which results in a heart attack. Sodium is salt. Adults should aim to consume less than 2400 mg of sodium per day. This includes table salt and salt added to food. If you have diabetes, you are advised to consume even less salt. Fresh foods generally contain much less salt than the packaged foods.

TOTAL CARBOHYDRATES

The total carbohydrates that you see in the label includes sugars, dietary fibers and other carbohydrates. Carbohydrates are part of a balanced and healthy diet. However, there are some carbohydrates that are better than others. Try to get most of your carbohydrates from sources such as fruits, vegetables, beans and whole grains.

Sugars that you see on food labels include both added sugars and natural. Added sugars are found in products such as soft drinks and cookies while natural sugars are found in fruit and milk. Limit your consumption of added sugars. You can do this by consulting the list of ingredients shown at the bottom of the label. Added sugar names appearing in labels include:

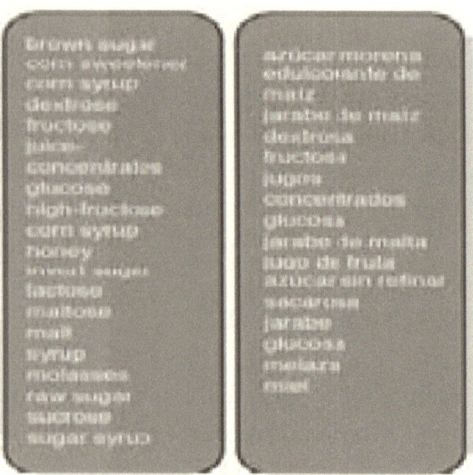

PROTEIN

Protein helps develop muscles. Foods like chicken, tofu, seafood, nuts and beans have a high content of protein.

INGREDIENTS

As a general rule, the fewer ingredients a product has the healthier it will be. Our bodies evolved over millions of years, feeding on the wealth of nature and that is what most favors it. The ingredients are presented in descending order, maximum amount to the minimum amount. This means that foods that label sugar in first or second place on the list have a higher sugar content and a low content of other nutrients.

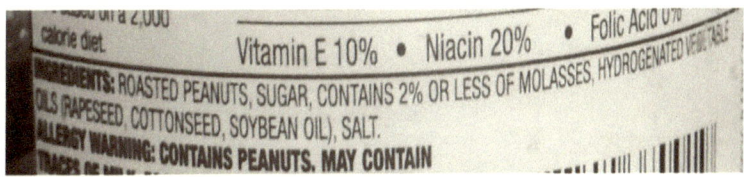

FASHION TERMS: REDUCED FAT, LOW-FAT AND LIGHT

Don't let these words make you think automatically that these products are healthy. These terms are often used on packets to describe products that may have low fat but it may not necessarily mean they are nutritious. A low-fat food may also have high sugar or calories and not offer much benefit.

{The healthiest food will always be those with a single ingredient.}

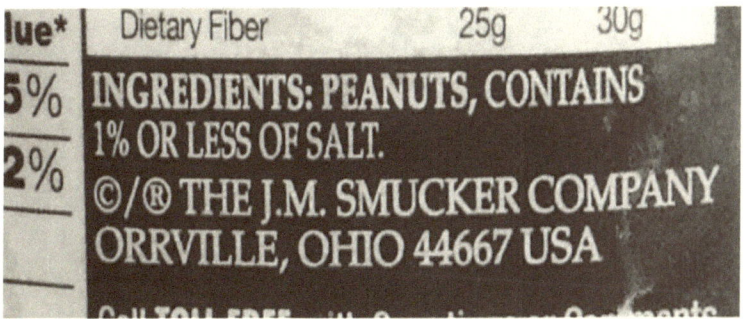

Ingredients: Sugar, enriched flour (wheat flour, niacin, reduced iron, thiamine mononitrate, riboflavin, folic acid), peanuts, vegetable shortening (palm, partially hydrogenated palm kernel, and/or cottonseed oils), contains less than 2% of: cocoa (processed with alkali), high fructose corn syrup, corn syrup solids, leavening (sodium bicarbonate, monocalcium phosphate, ammonium bicarbonate), salt, soy lecithin, natural and artificial flavor, artificial color (red #40 lake, yellow #5 lake, blue #1 lake, blue #2 lake).

Contains: Wheat, soy, peanuts.

ALLERGEN INFORMATION: This product is manufactured on equipment that processes products containing milk and coconut.

NUTS, THE MOST NUTRITIOUS AND HEALTHY FOOD

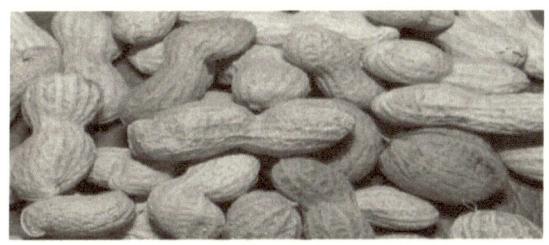

Walnuts contain more and better antioxidants than other fruits with a shell or skin.

Studies have shown that dried fruits, particularly those with a hard shell, are very nutritious and good for your health, particularly for heart health.

New research, focused on nuts with hard shells, found that the nut is a natural product "almost perfect" because of its high level of antioxidants and proteins.

Related stories

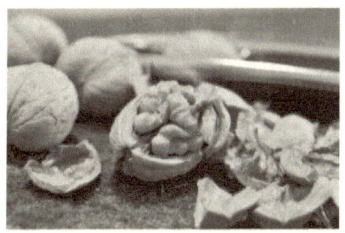

- Nuts help to lower cholesterol
- Good food for the heart

In addition to its nutritional benefits, these products contain high levels of polyphenols, antioxidant chemical compounds that help the body fight the effects of molecules that cause oxidation and damage to cells.

Past studies suggest that regular consumption of these dry fruits can reduce the risk of cardiovascular disease, certain cancers and type 2 diabetes.

More and Better Antioxidants

According to scientists at the University of Scranton, Pennsylvania, among hard-shelled dry fruits, nuts contain a greater combination of antioxidants in number and greater quality than any of them.

The study, which was presented at the Annual Meeting of the United States Chemical Society, analyzed nutrient levels of nine types of hard shell nuts: walnuts, pistachios, almonds, peanuts, Brazil nuts, pine nuts, cashews, macadamias and pecans.

"A handful of nuts contain almost twice as much antioxidants than an equivalent amount of other dry hard-shelled fruit that is commonly consumed."

All these products are rich in nutrients like vitamin E, minerals, and monounsaturated fatty acids and polyunsaturated.

The scientists found that walnuts contain more antioxidant polyphenols than any other fruit.

"We found that it is above peanuts, almonds, pecans, pistachios and other nuts."

"But unfortunately, people do not eat enough nuts. And this study shows that you should eat more of this product as part of a healthy diet," adds the researcher.

"Good" fats, nuts not only contain more antioxidants than other dry fruits, but also the antioxidants they have are much more powerful and potent.

For example, polyphenol antioxidants of nuts are between four and 15 times more potent than vitamin E, which is known to be very beneficial for its powerful antioxidant effects.

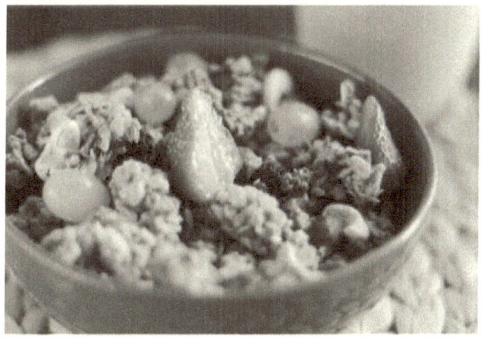

The study analyzed the level of antioxidants of nine different types of dry fruits.

Another advantage to choosing nuts as a source of antioxidant, "The heat released by roasting the fruit usually reduces the quality of its antioxidants" "People eat raw and unroasted nuts, and so you get all the effectiveness of these compounds," he adds.

A mistaken belief about these products, it is thought that if you eat large amounts of them then you'll get fat because its high calorie and fat content.

"Nuts contain polyunsaturated fats and monounsaturated, these are 'good fats' and do not contain harmful saturated fats that can cause narrowing of the arteries."

And to complete its benefits as an "almost perfect" food, nuts are a great source of protein and high quality, which according to researchers, it can be substituted for meat, and are full of vitamins, minerals, fiber, and are free of lactose and gluten. Just eat some seven nuts a day to get all the potential health benefits of these products.

Thank you to all who helped out with this book and for giving me ideas: Cristina Lazaro de Palibrio for your patience and great Help / a Yahilily Garcia for your support and contribution to the photos of my three decades / Wilmer Valencia for the cover photo and back cover of the book /Jhiael Otero Arraez editing food Pyramid/ Mark Barnes for the translation from Spanish to English, my family and ever-present friends in the whole process. And our God, my Heavenly Father for his hand touching this book for the benefit of His children and their own temples, who is you, reading this book.

Thanks to My Friend Gary Samuelson share this messages:

> "Through years of scientific studies we are constantly gaining a better understand the physical laws that govern the correct function of our body. On the most basic level, we require, oxygen, nutrition, hydration, sleep and exercise. I would like to thank Asdrubal for writing a book with a wealth of information and motivation for proper nutrition of our living machine, a machine that is built to run on the foods that nature provides. May we all learn these lessons and enjoy greater health."
>
> Thanks,
> -Gary Samuelson

D77=. Samuelson was awarded his Ph.D. in Atomic/ Medical Physics from the University of Utah and has received the American Association of Physics Teachers Award for Teaching Excellence. He works as an independent science consultant

Email to drubinlife coment about the book June -2 -2015

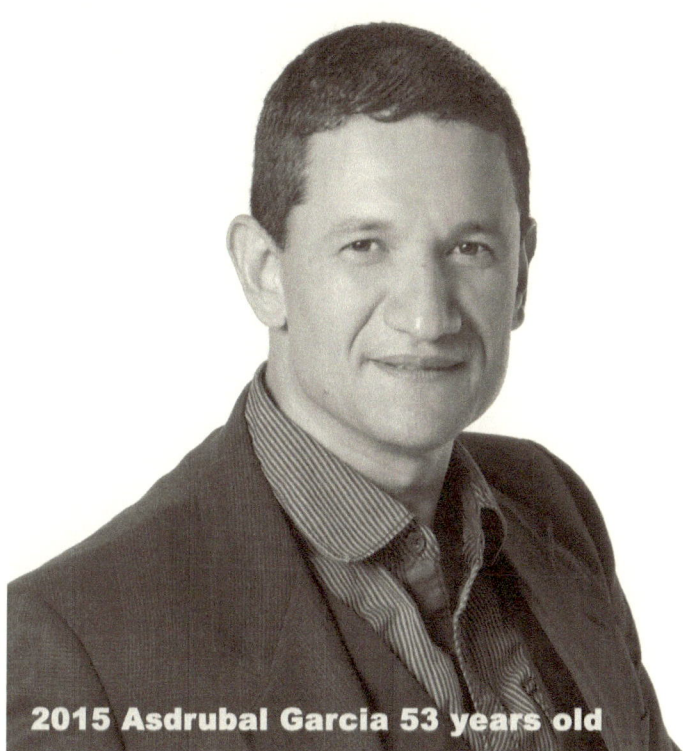
2015 Asdrubal Garcia 53 years old